The Anti-Medicine

Eating to Live Without Disease

PART 1

by Albert Mosséri

INDEX

Chapter 1: Waiting For Hunger 03
Chapter 2: Healthy Stools 17
Chapter 3: The Time Required for Digestion 19
Chapter 4: Coffee, Tea and Sal 25
Chapter 5: Starch 26
Chapter 6: Supplements 29
Chapter 7: Fresh Frui 31
Chapter 8: Dried Fruit 39
Chapter 9: Greens and Raw Vegetables 43
Chapter 10: Vegetables and Root Vegetables 47
Chapter 11: Nuts and Seeds 50
Chapter 12: Cheese 53
Chapter 13: Milk 56
Chapter 14: Chapter Meat, Fish and Bread 58
Chapter 15: Combining Bad Foods 61
Chapter 16: What's Important and What's Secondary 66
Chapter 17: Natural Combinations 71
Chapter 18: The Natural Hygiene System 77

Eating to Live Without Disease   by Albert Mosséri

CHAPTER 1: Waiting For Hunger

What's the point of reaching for pears for when we're thirsty if we don't know how to save onto our thirst for pears? Prof. Edouard Roux

We can appropriate the quote if we replace the word "thirst" with the word "hunger."

Thus, we would read: what's the point reaching for pears for when we're hungry if we don't know how to save our hunger for pears?

The word "hunger" is used to designate two different things:

1. **A state of deprivation, starvation, poverty or deficiency.** This type of hunger is a problem which results in malnutrition and various diseases, deficiencies and illnesses which do not typically exist in affluent countries.

2. **A state in which an individual feels the need to eat.** It is the expression of the same bodily instincts that are evidence of a healthy and vigorous life.

Hunger should guide our food practices, not be absent from them. It's the only thing that warns us of our need to eat.

Without it, we would be going through life like a plane without a pilot. Why? We would give our body food when it doesn't need it. The body is unable to benefit from this excess food, and therefore, it will eventually become overburdened.

Imagine giving water to a plant that doesn't need water. The excess of water will eventually cause the plant to suffer or even die. Similarly, cars have many indicator lights which warn drivers about many things. Needles, dials, and signals are there to inform the driver that the motor is too hot or that the car needs water, gasoline, or oil. Without this guidance, the car would fall apart. If these signals are unheeded and the car continues along its route, it would undoubtedly be at the center of several accidents. No pilot would fly without knowing where they are going. Knowing where they are going is the only guarantee that they will arrive.

Similarly, hunger is also our only guarantee of providing our body with what it needs at precisely the right moment. It is an invaluable guide. We must turn to it for guidance rather than ignore it. We must follow it and respect its instructions. In the end, we will reap the rewards.

Learning to Listen to Yourself

We must learn pay attention to and correctly interpret our feelings. They are the guiding force in our life, insofar as they are still reliable and neither perverted nor degraded.

For example, smokers often find it difficult to appreciate the flavor of fruit because tobacco has blunted their natural sense of smell.

Here's a more compelling case. People whose stomach is irritated by proteins, strong spices, coffee or wine often imagine that they are hungry after consuming these foods. However, this irritation is nothing more than a false sense of hunger which we can, with a bit of discernment, distinguish from true hunger.

Thus, if we ignore our instincts or we don't correctly understand them, we risk our health.

Therefore, we must be able to differentiate between real hunger and the false hunger we have only just begun to discuss.

When we taste a morsel of food and find it to be bitter or spicy, acrid or repulsive, it's a warning sign from our instincts, warning us not to continue eating it.

When we're tired, we experience physical sensations which lead us to rest by telling us to stop for a moment. These feelings tell us not to stimulate ourselves by drinking coffee or another form of "pick-me-up." When we do the opposite to pursue work or some other activity, we draw upon our body's reserves while simultaneously poisoning it. Coffee, for example, contains more than 15 toxins!

We must patiently learn the language of our various feelings, just as we would do in learning Spanish or German.

Avoiding Stimulation

As we have just discussed, we mustn't deceive ourselves by using stimulants, no matter how innocuous they may seem.

In fact, stimulation is nothing more than a myth — an illusion.

When we drink a cup of coffee in the morning, we imagine that it is helping us regain our strength and wake up while in reality, it drains us.

When we consume pepper or salt, we often imagine that we are hungry. In fact, these substances are poisoning us.

When we use laxatives, we are mostly beating our intestines and forcing them to work, thereby further exhausting them, when we should be looking for the cause of the problem (bread, grains, cheese).

Also, Avoid Simulation

(Not to be confused with *stimulation*)

We also mustn't seek to simulate slow natural functions through the use of means which are, in the end, harmful and deceptive.

We mustn't seek to stimulate nor simulate hunger by using seasonings to provoke the false hunger we discussed above.

False hunger is nothing more than an ersatz — a meaningless imitation.

We must learn to listen to our feelings. They are our best guides in life. We must respect them rather than mislead, betray and distort them with grotesque simulations that are simply imitations of the functions they seek to replace.

For example, laxative-induced diarrhea from drugs has nothing to do with the normal functioning of peristalsis.

The stupor provoked by sleeping pills has nothing do with restorative sleep.

Stimulation with coffee has nothing to do with the euphoric state of consciousness which stems from abundant energy.

False hunger has nothing to do with the real hunger that reflects our body's need for food.

Stomach Contractions

Some people feel stomach contractions at regular intervals during their regular meal hours.

"The idea that the sensation of being hungry is due to these contractions should be permanently abandoned," Shelton affirms.

"In fact, we have observed that individuals who have had their stomach removed always feel hungry. We removed the stomach of several rodents, and we noted that they were also always hungry, searching for food and eating. This study confirms that stomach contractions are not the cause of hunger.

Two American physiologists, Cannon and Carlson, have researched hunger and have carried out a series of experiments. They inserted a rubber balloon into the stomach which was connected to a tube that inflated the balloon from the outside when it reaches the stomach. Through this experiment, they were able to observe and measure the force of stomach contractions. They noted that the contractions were more intense at meal times, but they concluded, rather hastily, that these contractions provoked hunger.

They also found that hunger could be present without the presence of these contractions and vice versa. This last observation ought to have prevented them from jumping to any hasty conclusions. This was their mistake!

"As a notorious physiologist," Shelton rightly points out, "the famous Professor Carlson should have suspected that the stomach, sensing the presence of a foreign body (the balloon), was trying to reject it, especially when the balloon was inflated. Thus, the effort exerted by the stomach became frantic.

"Unable to reject the balloon during its first attempt, the stomach then rested to begin the process again later with increased contractions, in hopes of dislodging the foreign body. If these contractions then became painful due to their intensity as the stomach tried to reject the intruder, that pain had nothing to do with the normal stomach contractions that occur rhythmically around periods of hunger.

"The logical place to study the sensation of hunger is not in a laboratory, where experimental abnormalities are deliberately produced. It is among healthy, hungry people.

"That is why those who have monitored many fasts and had many opportunities to observe the manifestations of hunger are in a better position to describe it than physiologists in a lab. Professor Carlson certainly acknowledged this fact. He even did a short fast himself to study hunger, but his period of fasting was too short to eliminate unusual symptoms which he had presumed to be hunger."

A Delicious Sensation

We followed approximately three thousand people who were fasting. When detoxification decreases substantially through the depletion of vital reserves, weight becomes stable. Breath becomes less foul smelling, urine becomes clear, the mind and ideas become clear, and the person becomes optimistic and euphoric.

Hunger is sometimes felt like an "emptiness" in the stomach which then rises to the esophagus and mouth which respond by dilating and filling with saliva from glands squirting under the tongue on both sides. There is no pain, headache or painful sensation. Instead, it is a pleasant and delicious feeling.

Unpleasant or painful sensations in the stomach or head, tightness, stomach pain, or stomach cramps. These symptoms are not signs of hunger, but symptoms of gastritis, i.e., inflammation and congestion of the stomach's mucous membranes caused either by irritants (pepper, salt, condiments, coffee, wine) or by food indigestion.

When We Feel Our Organs

A person in good health will not feel his liver nor his stomach nor his colon nor any other organ in his body. When a person becomes aware of one of their organs, it's a sign of inflammation.

Congestion is part of the body's efforts to eliminate toxins from an inflamed area.

None of this has anything to do with hunger whose sensations should be delicious, not painful.

Graham, one of the pioneers of the Natural Hygiene movement, emphasized the following principle in his Lectures on the Science of Human Life:

> "When we become aware that we have a stomach, a liver or any other organ due to a sensation within that organ, we can be sure that something is not right.
>
> "In fact, as we have often said, when we are in good health, we shouldn't be aware of the existence of each of our organs, except basic needs which require us to exercise voluntary forces. Examples of this include our need to supply the body with food, our need to drink and our need to breathe air, as well as voluntary urination and bowel movements."

Therefore, we should never be aware of a healthy stomach, liver or kidneys. A sick stomach, liver or kidneys, on the other hand, will always be felt.

Pain and all other unpleasant stomach sensations are nothing more than morbid symptoms of an illness and will disappear if we abstain from eating for a few hours, sometimes a few days but rarely more.

We once had a client who suffered for seven consecutive days from atrocious burning in his stomach and esophagus. He abstained from eating and rested, and at the end of those seven days, everything returned to normal. We must not yield to the temptation to eat in conditions such as his to obtain relief. Palliation does not equate recovery.

We Must Choose the Best Moment

"Digestion," writes Shelton, "is one of life's greatest labors. Therefore, it follows that we should determine the best conditions in which to eat, as well as the best way to eat so that the digestive process can proceed without facing any obstacles.

"A person who eats when they aren't hungry won't digest their food as well as if they were to eat only when they were hungry. An individual who eats a sandwich rapidly or "on the go" as we say, won't benefit from the meal. The sandwich will pass the next day in a large, loose and foul-smelling bowel movement, accompanied by gas.

"Life is not a continuous feast. Even after ingesting the best foods in the world, if they weren't eaten in a favorable atmosphere which supports their digestion, the person eating them will not receive their money's worth from the meal. If you quickly swallow your food instead of properly chewing it, if you eat while feeling angry or afraid, if you are concerned or anxious, if you aren't serene and relaxed at the table, if you are surrounded by agitation, argument or discussion, if you are tired, feverish or in pain…all of these situations can prevent your food from being properly processed by your digestive enzymes.

"It's obvious that in situations such as these, hunger can't exist. In fact, fatigue prevents hunger; worries, quarrels, fears, fevers, and pain also prevent hunger. We commonly say that emotional distress prevents hunger.

"When you take time to taste your food, it helps with digestion. It is therefore essential that eating gives us real pleasure. In fact, if we were to derive the utmost pleasure from every meal we consume over the course of our lifetime, we would derive more pleasure from food than from any other activity.

"Unlike other sources of pleasure, neither age, failure, nor loneliness has the power to prevent you from enjoying this exquisite pleasure. Thus, it is imperative that you get the maximum satisfaction from what you eat.

"Every minute at the table is worth its weight in gold. Each delicate bite of food should fill us with ease. Each succulent morsel of natural foods should satisfy us."

We know that a relaxed atmosphere is conducive to procuring the maximum amount of pleasure from a meal. We don't imagine feasts as taking place in a climate of tension, anger, and heated discussion!

Nevertheless, we don't know that rushing, hastiness, temperature, and pain are an obstacle to digestion nor that we mustn't eat in these conditions.

Unfortunately, feasts bring us more mental than physical pleasure with their various mixtures, various tastes, delicately prepared dishes and their pleasant company. We try to make the most of it without paying too heavy a price by gorging ourselves on a minimal number of samples.

On the other hand, hunger is the essential condition for enjoying what we eat, though it would certainly be agreeable to eat with those whom we love and cherish due to the relaxation and serenity their presence provides.

Lastly, talking while eating prevents us from properly chewing our food. It's a bad habit that we must eliminate. It's fine to exchange a few pleasantries, but it's unacceptable to carry on a prolonged conversation.

How to Be Hungry

"When we are unable to derive the utmost satisfaction in what we are eating, it might as well be a commandment to fast! Fasting should last until we are once again able to find this pleasure."

"We mustn't be afraid to fast. Before it does us any harm, we will become so ravenous that we will be unable to resist eating."

It should go without saying that we should eat foods as Nature has given them to us, without preparation, seasonings, and additives.

It must be noted, however, that there is a critical limitation to fasting which only a competent professional hygienist can recognize.

The return of true hunger in an otherwise healthy person who has detoxified their body through a fast should be a flawless, automatic process.

Unfortunately, this instinct is often depraved and perverted. Its mechanisms have become disorganized and dysfunctional. This is why we use other signs to tell ourselves to stop fasting: the stabilization of weight for three days on two separate occasions. When such a fast is followed by a detox diet, hunger will bloom like a late rose.

An Interesting Case

A 51-year-old woman had been fasting under my care for 33 days with neither problem nor crisis, except for diarrhea which lasted for several days.

On the night of the 33rd day, around 9 o'clock, she began to feel real hunger. At 10 o'clock in the evening, she called me:

"What are you feeling?"

"Real hunger," she told me, but I wasn't satisfied with her response. I wanted details.

"What exactly are you feeling?"

"It's a sucking feeling starting at the bottom of my gut, moving toward my stomach and my esophagus, toward my mouth."

It was perfect. It was true hunger. We stopped her fast and fed her a small apple, six times a day.

I am always wary when someone who is fasting tells me that their mouth is watering because it leads me to suspect that the person is simply repeating the symptoms of hunger they read in books, but this woman had a bad taste in her mouth during her entire fast. Her mouth tasted salty and horrid, but this disappeared near the end.

Currently, I no longer push fasting to these extremes. I follow a semi-fast which I call an elimination diet once my weight stabilizes three days on two separate occasions.

In Conclusion

According to Shelton, our number one rule is simple: "only eat when you are hungry."

Instead, I would say in a more positive way of thinking: wait until you're hungry to eat.

Of course, this way of phrasing amounts to the same idea, but I find that the idea of waiting, much like the concept of hope, is more positive to consider than abstention.

Men of the Past

"As for man, he mixes his foods regardless of where they originated.

"He combines the diet of carnivorous tigers, omnivorous squirrels, sheep, granivorous birds and fruitarian primates in a single meal.

Nevertheless, he believes that such a mixture of different foods will be digested as well and as quickly in his stomach, the as tiger's diet would be digested in the stomach of a sheep.

"Regardless of the human digestive tract's ability to adapt and adjust, it is not able to simultaneously adjust its digestive secretions to so many different types of diet at once.

"Why should we expect the human digestive tract to be able to process such mixtures?

"It has been argued that the human gastrointestinal tract has faced such mixtures for centuries "without a hitch," but such a declaration is not based upon fact but upon our ignorance about the history of human nutritive practices and the realities of contemporary human suffering.

"Current dietary habits are not even several centuries old. Until recently, man's meals included only two or three foods, and they were very simple. With several notable exceptions, even the meals of wealthy classes were simple compared to current dietary practices.

"Every student of humanity's diet knows that Americans are currently very modern and that the indiscriminate mixing of all kinds of foods in the stomach was not practiced in the past as we see it today.

"The further we delve into the study of our ancestors' food practices the simpler they appear to be.

"We know from everyday experience that simple meals are easier to digest.

"To say that our digestive tracts face such mixtures "without a hitch" is simply not true. It is apparent that this "hitch" has the proportions of a complaint on a national scale. Sodium bicarbonate or another similar medication has become our favorite dessert. Every year, we spend millions to alleviate the discomfort that typically follows our meals.

"When we observe the feeding practices of lower animals, we see the greatest simplicity.

"Each animal is limited to one kind of food: grass is the food of one species, fish is the food of another, animal flesh is the food of a third… Confine yourself to one food per meal, and when attempting to make this choice, consult your palate."

The Balanced Diet: a Myth

The medical notion of a balanced menu is a mistake. Nowhere in Nature do we find balanced diets. Neither cows, gorillas nor horses eat balanced diets.

Followers of "Instinctive Eating" have committed the same medical error. They will eat incompatible foods if their perverted sense of smell pushes them to do so.

As I pointed out at the beginning of this chapter, wild animals (not those that have been domesticated and fed by humans) tend to eat only one food per meal.

Even those who do eat a variety of foods tend to compose each meal of a single food. "Regardless of the human digestive tract's ability to adapt and adjust, it is not able to simultaneously adjust its digestive secretions to so many different types of diet at once.

"Why should we expect the human digestive tract to be able to process such mixtures?

Mono-Eating

Our predecessors in the pursuit of Natural Hygiene often avoided food incompatibilities by recommending that we eat only one type of food per meal.

Nevertheless, they simultaneously tried to discover possible harmonies between various foods through daily experimentation.

In this field, as in many others, we cannot say that we know everything. The truth is always changing. Over time, more knowledge will be revealed.

It is important not to be content with what we know and to open our minds to any and all future research. Once we sort through them, we will surely find the truth among all the far-fetched ideas.

With that being said, people who insist on eating one food per meal do have much to their credit. It is true that the human digestive tract, like that of lower animals, is better able to adjust its digestive juices to the nature of the food consumed if we only eat one variety at time.

Will the civilized man of the 21st century, whose mind has become sophisticated and who tastes food with his palate as much as with his brain and his imagination, be able to return to and be satisfied with simple menus limited to a single food, like pigeons, dogs, and snakes?

This is a tricky question.

For this reason, I believe it is essential for us to derive the maximum amount pleasure possible from what we eat with a minimal amount of accompanying problems. This is why we can tolerate compatible fruit mixtures and concordant vegetable mixtures. It is rare that two of these foods would be entirely incompatible.

Watch Out for Indigestible Combinations

"A little while ago," Shelton wrote, "I was at a friend's house. Several of us were watching TV ads"

"One of the advertisements featured a young boy topping bowl of cereal with two spoonfuls of white sugar, a sliced banana, a handful of raisins and a lot of milk.

"While he demonstrated his breakfast concoction, he rambled on and tried to convince the audience that this mixture was both tasty and nutritious.

"At the end, a young man that was watching the commercial made the following remark:

"Whenever I eat breakfast like that, I always have heartburn."

"You and several million others like you," I immediately added.

In fact, no digestive system in the world is suited to digest this kind of meal.

Any animal in nature would never eat such a diverse mix of foods.

It doesn't bode well for human intelligence that millions of men, women, and children continue to eat such indigestible combinations of food day after day and take medicines to alleviate the discomfort that ensues.

Every year, we spend millions of dollars buying drugs to treat the stomach acidity and gastric discomfort that are almost inevitable after eating a meal like this.

How to Tell If a Combination is Bad?

Obviously, every person won't have the digestive problems that Shelton describes. Each person's experience will vary depending on their genetics.

The next day, however, all of them will experience smelly and bulky stools, diarrhea or constipation and messy stools that require an excessive use of toilet paper. Furthermore, these bowel movements will be accompanied by foul-smelling gas. This is a tell-tale sign that the person ate an indigestible mixture the day before.

Shelton cites several digestive drugs, all containing sodium bicarbonate: Alka-Seltzer, Tums, Pepto-Bismol, Rolaids, etc. In addition to these patented medications, many people still use an old remedy of yesteryear: baking soda. Others use milk of magnesia. These drugs, which also produce their problems, specific to their application, provide foolish people with a semblance of temporary relief from discomfort caused by indigestion.

These medications have the biggest impact on the kidneys that are responsible for eliminating them from the body. Wouldn't it be wiser to just induce vomiting by tickling the throat like the Romans used to do after their meals?

The concoction that Shelton had seen on TV reminds me of Dr. Bircher Benner's muesli in Switzerland. It includes, even more, ingredients and indigestible mixtures.

"In the face of the unnecessary daily suffering of millions of people and the outrageous prices they pay for relief, how can we refuse to eat meals without incompatible food mixtures in exchange for avoiding all of these troubles?

"Everything we're saying about food compatibility is so simple that any person, regardless of technical training, could do it. There's no need to run experiments in laboratories. You can try it out at home by eating compatible meals by the rules established in our books and taking notes on the results. We can then compare these results with the results of your previous diet when you ate any and all food mixtures, pell-mell."

Testimonials

"One of my distributors recently sent me a photocopy of a letter he received from a woman in Pennsylvania who bought a copy of my book on food combinations. Here are some excerpts from that letter:

"I don't usually write letters of admiration, but this letter is more than that.

"In fact, it is a letter of appreciation, gratitude, and thanks.

"It was a happy day when I ordered your book on food combinations, written by Shelton. For years, I have suffered from indigestion, gas, bloating, discomfort and pain.

"Now, I try to combine food properly, and I no longer have any heartburn. No more gas, no bloating, no need for Alka-Seltzer, no baking soda, nothing. Why don't more people try this simple method? It must be that they don't know it exists."

"I have received," Shelton writes, "many letters like this one. Several people have written to me to confirm the same fact personally. Many of my readers say that they experienced relief after their first compatible meal.

"Just recently, a young man shared his experience with me. He told me that his whole family had been freed from their usual afternoon discomfort by eating only compatible foods. He and his family also found that they no longer needed drugs. Others had told me about how their so-called allergies disappeared when they learned how to eat compatible foods.

In my experience, bloating and gas are both caused consuming foods containing protein, such as nuts and cheeses. It is better to remove these foods from your diet and not attempt to combine them with other compatible foods.

Warning: Whether compatible or not, when we eat various nuts or cheeses, we will have bloating, heaviness, gas and bad stool the following day.

"Nature did not design the human digestive system to digest numerous and complicated meals..."

"Meals composed 7 or even 21 kinds of food were not a part of nature's design for the human digestive system.

Any person who sits down for a meal and eats several food mixtures, from cheese soup to pears and other fruits, is sure to suffer from indigestion. If that person then becomes accustomed to eating such complicated meals and ignoring the boundaries of his enzymes, as is often the case, this abdominal discomfort will become chronic. The person will always supply of pills in his pockets which he takes everywhere he goes. This habit of taking pills everywhere you go is certainly encouraged by the drug manufacturer.

This implies that it is more important for people to have a fictitious form of relief at hand than to simply learn how to eat healthily and eliminate the need for such alleviation. Is it that important for us to give money to drug manufacturers, at the expense of our health?

Digestive Aids

Before ending this chapter, I would like to share one last note regarding drugs that are supposed to help with digestion.

No medication can facilitate digestion, per se, because digestion is carried out by the digestive juices we secrete and by nothing else. We cannot force our glands to secrete these juices if they refuse to obey.

So, how do these medications alleviate the problems caused by indigestion? They just neutralize the acidity that indigestion produces.

The body must subsequently eliminate the "neutralized" food bolus, just as it must detox the drugs themselves. These drugs are chemical products.

In the end, this elimination exhausts both the liver and the kidneys by imposing a heavy burden upon them, i.e., liver or kidney disease.

We mustn't forget that these so-called diseases are our body's efforts to eliminate these substances.

CHAPTER 2: Healthy Stools

Healthy people who properly digest what they eat should have stools that:

1) are formed
2) are not stinky
3) aren't messy (not requiring excessive use of toilet paper)
4) are passed quickly

In an age where cleanliness is a national virtue, who can boast that they have odorless stools?

Who can boast of being clean, both inside and out?

We use perfumed soaps, colognes, and deodorants, and we wash every day of the year; we pride ourselves on being both clean and presentable.

This is only our appearance. It's nothing more than smoke and mirrors. It's as though we believe that everything that we're hiding and concealing isn't there. What rubbish!

The human digestive system is almost universally in a septic state. This means that fermentation and putrefaction have become so widespread that almost everyone suffers from putrescence in the stomach, intestines, and colon.

Evidence of this putrescence exists in most people in the form of bloating, gas, gurgling in the stomach, discomfort, foul-smelling stools, fetid breath, a coated tongue and a plethora of other marked symptoms.

The millions of dollars we spend annually on medications to compensate for these disorders are only further proof of humanity's general failure about its digestive functions.

Bulky stools signify that little to no food has been properly digested by the body.

Unformed, more or less liquid and inconsistent stools with roughly the same consistency as porridge indicate that the body has not had enough time to digest the food bolus in question and has rejected the bolus as is.

These stools often smear and require an excessive use of toilet paper.

Constipation often indicates that we have eaten cheese, bread or both.

Lastly, foul-smelling stools indicate that fermentation and putrefaction have turned the food bolus into stinking, poisonous trash.

"Indigestion has several causes: eating when you are upset, agitated, tired or uncomfortable, eating when you are in pain, have a fever or have inflammation, eating just before you do arduous physical labor or just before swimming in the sea can all lead to indigestion."

When you drink an ice-cold beverage or have an ice cream for dessert, it stops the digestive process because it must take place at body temperature. This results in both indigestion and diarrhea.

CHAPTER 3: The Time Required for Digestion

How long does it take for food to be completely and digested?

Digestion includes the consumption of food through the mouth, storage of food in the colon and the food's ultimate ejection from the body in the form of waste.

How long does this process take? Fifteen to twenty hours in total.

When books say that potatoes are digested in fifteen minutes, fruits in twenty minutes, cheese and meats in three hours, and nuts in four hours, they are only referring to the phases of digestion that occur in the stomach. The digestion processes that take place in the stomach require the most energy.

Because the stages of digestion which occurs in the stomach require the most energy, taking between one and four hours to complete, only the strongest events can affect digestion after this period.

Let's look at an example. Suppose you get up early in the morning and you receive some bad news about your professional situation, find out about the death of a dear relative or experience some other tragedy that knocks you off your feet. Any violent emotion that you might feel in these circumstances could lead to immediate intestinal disturbance or diarrhea.

Even if you had yet to eat anything that day, your emotions could cause the already digested food bolus you had consumed the day before to be rejected.

This proves that even a dozen hours aren't enough to fully process food.

It is also worth noting that diarrhea can occur almost immediately in extremely anxious people when they experience an intense emotion. It can even be brought on by a mere disturbance, anxiety or doubt. This is rather similar to babies, who typically pass stool shortly after eating.

Diarrhea or Vomiting? It Depends On Your Vitality

When you eat spoiled food or experience a detrimental event or violent emotion that knocks you off your feet, any digestion which may have been in progress for fifteen hours at the time of the stressful event will be interrupted.

This can result in diarrhea or, as we will soon see, other bodily reactions.

Why? The body functions like a computer or, depending on your perspective, computers function just like our the body. Both of these systems require energy to work. If you shut off your computer's power, it will stop working; your body functions in the same way. When you feel a strong emotion, your mind begins to monopolize all available energy to solve the problem that has arisen. After that, there is no more energy left for digestion.

There are several chemical stages in digestion. The first prepares the food for the second, the second for the third, and so on. If anyone of these steps lacks energy, the necessary chemical reactions can't occur, and digestion will be compromised. The bolus will then ferment and become diarrhea.

However, although I just said that it would become diarrhea, that's not always the case. Occasionally, it leads to vomiting.

Let's discuss this curious phenomenon. If you are in good health and have an abundance of energy, any spoiled foods will be spotted quickly by your physical senses and will be rejected as soon as they enter the stomach.

However, if you have bad health, have little energy or are disturbed emotionally, your senses won't perceive the food that needs to be rejected until later. The reaction will be too late at this point, and the food bolus will be eliminated as diarrhea rather than vomit.

Therefore, it follows that vomiting is the result of good health whereas diarrhea is the product of mediocre health.

> "One of the most common causes of the digestive failure is our modern habit of mixing different foods in our stomach.
>
> The human digestive system, like that of many other animals, is not designed to digest such complex mixtures and meals composed of several different kinds of food.
>
> Simple meals, eaten in moderation, facilitate digestion. This is how people have nourished themselves for nearly all of human history.
>
> It is only recently that in certain parts of the world, people have begun to overwhelm their digestive system with a huge variety of food in a single meal. The state of continual decomposition discussed above is primarily due to these very standard incompatible food mixtures. Furthermore, the combination of starches and proteins in a single meal is the worst of all.
>
> Thus, the habit of eating hot dogs is nothing more than an extension of the practice of eating bread and potatoes with meat. If we went

> back to our old habit of eating starches and proteins separately, we would be pleasantly surprised by the results.
>
> Critics like to say that eating proteins and starches together in a single meal is perfectly acceptable since healthy people do it all the time.
>
> However, is it true that healthy people eat combinations of proteins and starches? If it were possible to find a truly healthy person who ate the same way as the rest of the world, we would have our answer, but where are these healthy people? There aren't any! Why? There are several reasons, and a lack of comprehension of incompatible foods is certainly among them."

We have a slightly different opinion than Shelton. We find that the combination of acid and starches is the worse.

As for eating proteins and starches together, if it never produces health problems, it's because the foods they consumed are not human-specific: meat and bread or nuts and bread, for example.

It's certainly not impossible to find relatively healthy people who occasionally eat incompatible food mixtures, but do they have odorless stools? That is the absolute test of a person's health. These seemingly healthy people will eventually accumulate rheumatic diseases and other illnesses. Rather than suffering as young adults, they will suffer from disease when they become elderly in the not-so-distant future.

> "It's true," Shelton admits, "that healthy people often eat starches and proteins together, but in reality, they live rather recklessly in every respect. They smoke, drink, overeat and make mistakes that are detrimental to their health.
>
> "These people will maintain that they are in excellent health, yet they will simultaneously emit the most foul-smelling gas in existence! They'll brush their teeth every morning to clean away the dirt and bad taste, yet they'll then smoke a cigarette to palliate their nerves.
>
> "We are accepting an extremely low level of health when we praise individuals such as these for being healthy.
>
> "Doctors often deny that there are food mixtures which can cause the decomposition of consumed foods. Then, they cite other doctors in their field to confirm their statements. They seem as though they're saying that their statements are true because they say their statements are true. As soon as medicine declares something through the voices of its many practitioners, it becomes truth!

"Asserting that harmful mixtures are good does not make them good. Asserting that medicine is correct or that those who eat pell-mell mixtures digest their good better does not make those facts true either.

"Yet, we cannot help noticing that those who insist on eating incompatible food mixtures are still palliating their illnesses with medications, but when they begin to eat compatible foods, they stop needing them altogether.

"Why is modern medicine less knowledgeable about digestion than any other human function?"

AND PHYSIOLOGISTS?

"Unfortunately, though it pains me to say it, physiologists almost never try to connect their discoveries with real life. The only connection they try to make is between physiological fact and the practice of medicine.

"This is not a sufficient reason for medicine's ignorance. It is nevertheless true that a few rare physicians make independent efforts to relate physiology to everyday life."

Shelton was only trying to say that when physiologists discover that acids stop the production of ptyalin in the mouth, for example, they don't put this discovery into practice by recommending that acids and starches be eaten separately.

Their support for these discoveries is purely theoretical. They never use what they learn to provide practical implications for everyday life.

"Prescribing pepsin, hydrochloric acid, baking soda, anodyne and other medications to palliate indigestion while ignoring its causes is not an intelligent practice.

"When illness and discomfort follow certain mixtures of incompatible foods, it is certainly easy to overcome it with drugs and deny that the combinations as mentioned above were ever involved.

"Thus, we continue to eat pell-mell and palliate our troubles by taking medications after each meal. We see this in millions of cases.

"Yet, an intelligent person will try to understand why they have discomfort that needs to be palliated in the first place. They will then realize that digestion isn't meant to be an unpleasant process and that acid reflux, bloating and colic are not typically associated with normal digestion. When authorities continue to belittle the notion of compatible foods as much as they want, we are forced to acknowledge their commercial motives.

The fact that medical authorities bash compatible foods and that the public goes along with them is due to the simple fact that practicing Natural Hygiene is an obstacle to succulent dishes, artificial flavors and elaborate meals prepared by highly qualified chefs. Upsetting consumers isn't good for the medical field, lest sick people abandon the practice altogether.

"A large salad made with raw vegetables (such as lettuce, cucumber, celery, etc.) and no tomatoes, two non-starchy, cooked vegetables, and protein: that's the kind of meal that will be easily digested and pose no problems to one's health. If we add bread, potatoes, milk, sugar, and fruit to this meal, digestion would be delayed, and pain would ensue.

"Authorities issue positive reports on food mixtures after saying that everyone mixes starches and proteins without problems and that Nature has seen fit to combine them in foods that it produces itself (such as grains). These same authorities nevertheless refuse to experiment with compatible foods, and as such, they aren't honest with themselves or the public.

"Why should we avoid mixing starchy foods with acids? Medical authorities agree that this is an acceptable mixture, and I'm sure that the manufacturers of Alka-Seltzer and Rolaids agree.

"Why should we avoid food combinations that lead to fermentation when we can quickly overcome these symptoms with medications? Why bother with complicated rules, when a simple pill can get you back on your feet in record time? Why avoid the causes of poor health, fragility, and mediocrity when we can just ease their symptoms with medications?

"We choose medication because of laziness, negligence, taste and a lack of discipline.

"It is a well-documented physiological fact that acids destroy salivary ptyalin (salivary amylase) and stop the salivary digestion of the starches.

"This interruption can be caused by acidic fruits, vinegar, or the hydrochloric acid contained in gastric juice.

"Indigestion may not produce any disturbance in so-called healthy stomachs, but if there is any pre-existing stomach irritation, the mixture will be intolerable

"We mustn't worry about the contrary opinion issued by the medical authorities when a simple test can give us incontestable proof of rule's correctness. All we must do is separate fruits and starches.

"Throw away your medications and eat compatible foods. This practice will keep you out of trouble.

"The way we digest fruit is so different from how we digest other foods that it is better to eat them alone rather than mix them with starches or proteins.

"Many doctors just condemn fruits entirely, saying that they disturb digestion, but this is only true when we eat them with starches, such as in a dessert. When eaten alone, fruits have a wealth of benefits." Vol. 31, No. 11, Dr. Shelton's Hygienic Review.

CHAPTER 4: Coffee, Tea and Salt

Even the most compatible foods can become indigestible if we consume them with toxic substances like coffee, tea, and salt.

"Coffee and tea inhibit the digestion of food in the stomach due to the toxic substances they contain and the sugars that often accompany them."

Perversely, people tend to believe that teas and many so-called digestive herbs can help facilitate digestion.

In reality, digestion is being confused with indigestion. When we consume these drinks, we immediately feel the effects of our body struggling to digest them (i.e., heaviness, sleepiness and bloating) because the dilution and inhibition of our gastric juices lead to total indigestion.

When we experience indigestion, we don't feel anything at first. The food bolus will pass through our body the following day, but it won't be properly digested or absorbed in our stools. As a result, the stools will be bulky, foul-smelling and unformed, and they will often be messy and stain the body.

"All kinds of condiments can also inhibit the digestion of food in the stomach because of the stomach irritation they cause.

"It's likely that they also inhibit intestinal digestion because they are indigestible and cause irritation all along the digestive tract."

"Salt is also guilty of inhibiting food digestion in the stomach.

"There are several diet products which are widely sold in stores that are made of powdered vegetables. Some of these products contain seaweed, which is very salty on its own, while other powders contain added salt. These products are used in soups, sprinkled on salads and other foods, used as seasonings and sometimes used as supplements. These can also inhibit digestion within the stomach, sometimes for hours."

Therefore, these substances can render even the most compatible foods indigestible.

CHAPTER 5: Starch

Before we discuss compatible starches in detail, let's look at some of their characteristics.

When we talk about starches or starchy foods, we're referring to grains and roots (potatoes, Jerusalem artichokes, rutabaga, sweet potato, taro, just to name a few).

Legumes are also starchy foods, but since they also contain a high percentage of protein, we won't be including them in our discussion.

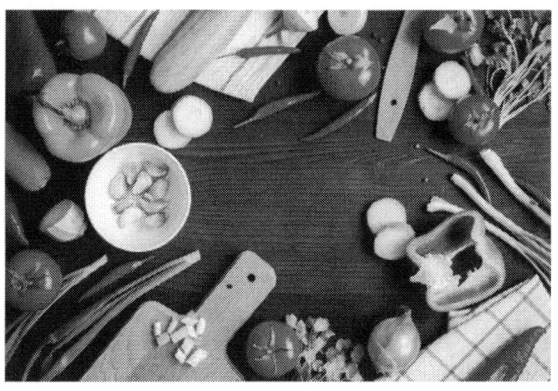

There are vegetables which contain a minimal amount of starch or simple sugars, like cauliflower, artichokes, green beans, cabbage, chard, and peppers.

"Carlton Fredericks," Shelton writes, "is considered to be the most qualified dietician in the United States. He was a biochemist who spent eight years working with Dr. Casimir Funk, the man who coined the term "vitamins" and was a pioneer in the field. Mr. Fredericks gave lectures on nutrition to thousands of doctors, dentists, and nurses. He was regularly invited to do radio broadcasts, and he wrote several books about nutrition.

"In other words, his authority was universally recognized.

"He established rules for consuming starches. In his opinion, people should eat no more than two starchy, sugary foods in a single meal.

"Therefore, if you were to have a meal that included both bread and potatoes, for example, you would have exhausted your starch allotment.

"A single meal," he says, "consisting of peas, bread, potatoes, sugars, and desserts should also include pills, vitamin B, sodium bicarbonate and the addresses of the nearest arthritis and degenerative disease specialists."

Fredericks was moving closer to the rules of Natural Hygiene, which tells us that we should consume a maximum of one carbohydrate per meal, rather than the two starches suggested by Fredericks.

But let's not forget that "carbohydrates" includes both starches and sugars.

Furthermore, this rule does not apply to foods that only contain small amounts of starches, such as those outlined above. Thus, we can consume mixtures of cauliflower, cabbage, green beans and so forth.

It's important to be able to distinguish between highly concentrated starchy foods, moderately starchy foods and foods with a relatively small amount of starch.

HIGHLY CONCENTRATED STARCHY FOODS

- Bread
- Grains, wheat, millet, corn, buckwheat, rice, etc.
- Legumes (dry peas, white beans, lentils, dried beans, chickpeas, soy)

MODERATELY STARCHY FOODS

- Potatoes
- Jerusalem artichokes
- Rutabaga
- Tapioca
- Yams
- Sweet potatoes
- Kohlrabi
- Parsnip

FOODS WITH LOW AMOUNTS OF STARCH

- Cauliflower
- Green beans
- Zucchini
- Carrots
- Celery

It's possible to mix foods with a low amount of starch in a single meal without experiencing problems. When it comes to moderately starchy foods, it's important to take care not to eat too many of them, but they can also be combined with other low to moderately starchy foods.

It is better to completely avoid highly concentrated starchy foods because they also contain a lot of protein.

Furthermore, highly concentrated starchy foods should not be mixed with other moderately to highly concentrated starchy foods.

For example, bread should not be combined with potatoes because the body tends to prioritize whichever food is easiest to digest. In this case, the potatoes would be digested first.

"For more than forty years," Sheldon writes, "the practice of Natural Hygiene has consisted of eating a large salad, without starches."

These salads appeared to be huge in relation the small quantities we would typically eat. They are made up of fresh, raw vegetables and contain significant amounts of vitamins and minerals in an authentic form (as opposed to dietary supplements such as capsules and yeast).

CHAPTER 6: Supplements

Let's digress for a moment to discuss the supplements available in health food stores.

"The only thing that can satisfy people who enjoy practicing Natural Hygiene is an authentic product in its natural state. It must be that or nothing at all," Shelton writes.

"Practitioners of Natural Hygiene refuse to take dietary supplements and anything else that that comes from a factory."

The purpose of nutritional supplements is purely commercial. They are a byproduct of our medicinal fetish and obsession with the medical notion of a cure, no matter how foolish it may be.

Fredericks, the renowned dietician we discussed above, recommended dietary supplements and emphasized the work done by the vitamins that they contain.

A large, raw salad provides our body with all of the elements it needs, whether currently known or as-of-yet undiscovered.

At any rate, taking dietary supplements and chemical substances doesn't solve the problem. They are of no use to the human body as it is incapable of assimilating them.

There is no better source for dietary substances than the vegetable kingdom. Chemists cannot create acceptable and natural foods.

Let's briefly return to our discussion of starches.

According to Fredericks, we can eat two starches in a single meal but no more. According to him, we could simultaneously eat bread and potatoes, for example, but we would have exhausted our starch allotment in doing so.

Practitioners of Natural Hygiene, on the other hand, suggest eating only one moderately to highly concentrated starchy food per meal for two reasons:

1) The body tends to digest whoever food is easiest and leaves the other to ferment.

2) Two moderately to highly starchy foods in a single meal is too much starch.

When I see baby food made up of five different grains, I find myself pitying the poor children.

This combination is wrong in itself, but even when eaten in isolation, grains are not meant for human consumption.

We only have to look at (and smell) the stools of these innocent young creatures to see that their food is also fermenting within them.

CHAPTER 7: Fresh Fruit

People with a weak digestive system will benefit from sticking to a single type of fresh fruit, eaten alone, even if they change the fruit every time they eat. They cannot allow themselves to eat several types of fruit in one sitting.

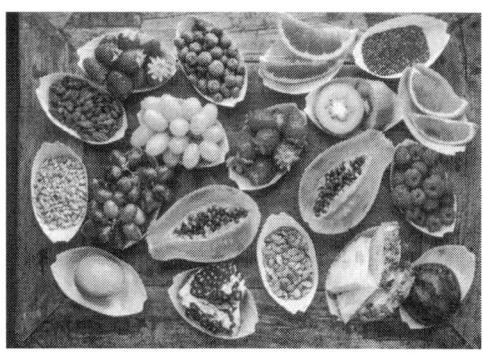

As for people with a stronger digestive system, they can eat several kinds of fruit at once. It is even preferable that they do so.

In fact, if a healthy person were to eat nothing but a lot of oranges, there is a chance that they could introduce too much acid into their body. If they are toxic, they will suffer from some enervation. If that person were to eat nothing but pears, it's possible that they wouldn't be able to digest them properly. If they were to eat nothing but grapefruit, they would quickly become fed up with the fruit which, on its own, is insufficient to nourish a person adequately. They can't limit themselves to peaches either as they are a natural diuretic.

If a person were to eat nothing but apples, on the other hand, they wouldn't suffer from any problems as a result, for they are the king of all fruits.

Nevertheless, a mixture of fruits mitigates the problems that a single variety of fruit can bring about when consumed alone. Furthermore, people are typically more satisfied with a meal when it is varied.

Monotony in Nature

It would seem that in nature, monotony is a rule of thumb. Dogs will always eat meat and horses will always eat grass without ever getting bored with their diet or calling for change. They carry themselves perfectly well.

Unfortunately, human beings must also satisfy their mind and imagination which have both become rather sophisticated. As civilization has developed, our ability to be satisfied with the simplicity of nature has disappeared.

This is why I'm not in favor of too much simplicity and monotony in meals, provided that variation is physiologically possible. However, we mustn't buy into overly sophisticated meals as we tend to do throughout our civilized society. These complicated meals don't nourish our bodies, even if they are extravagant to behold and captivate our imagination.

We can't only live by feeding our mind!

At a certain point, we must choose between illness and health.

Many people are not content with eating fruits as they are. Instead, they prefer to mix them in some salad, cutting them and artistically arranging them on a decorated plate as a landscaper might do with flower beds and the greenery that surrounds them.

Juices

What about juices? For beginners, juices are acceptable to satisfy their cravings, though some people see drinking juices as an elegant, almost snobbish gesture, that contrasts with the vulgarity of biting into an apple with your teeth, creating a noise that might shock chaste ears.

Nature, however, did not produce juices. They move through the digestive system too quickly for them to be digested properly, whereas when we consume whole fruits, digestion is much slower and efficient.

Therefore, the danger in drinking juices is that they can potentially lead to indigestion and fermentation, especially if they are swallowed in one gulp. They should be sipped slowly.

Furthermore, the pulp that we detest and push to the side contains all of the drink's precious nutrients. The so-called indigestible pulp cleans our intestines and prevents constipation. With that being said, there are, of course, situations in which we have no choice but to drink juice.

In conclusion, all fresh fruits are compatible with one another, except for bananas.

Acidic Fruits

Aside from citrus fruits, which we never eat in isolation, pineapples are the most acidic fruit we consume. There are also some rather acidic types of oranges.

Fruit, whether acidic or not, are compatible with one another and with other moderately acidic fruits.

The acids that these fruits contain are poisons that the body must eliminate to benefit from the other nutritious substances contained in the fruit. This elimination occurs with the help of the body's alkali. Nevertheless, following the digestion, fruit brings more to the body than it took.

On the other hand, if fruit is not well-digested, the second digestive phase can't take place, and the fruit remains acid-forming.

Fruits may not be adequately digested due to:

- The consumption of various nuts (almonds, hazelnuts, etc.), even if they were consumed at a different point in the day because these protein foods inhibit our digestive ability.
- Extreme fatigue during a meal.
- A bad food combination.
- A lack of hunger.
- A negative emotion.

Very ill people benefit from temporarily limiting their consumption of overly acidic fruits while their fragile health recovers a bit. They should eat more raw vegetables than fruit.

Fruits are not compatible with starches such as potatoes and cooked vegetables. In fact, their acidity destroys ptyalin, the salivary starch, thus stopping the digestion of the starches.

Should We Peel Our Fruits?

In general, fruit peels are indigestible and end up in the stools. Tomato skin is an obvious example of this. The same goes for grape, apple and pear skins. We can chew them for extended periods of time, and nothing will happen. Chewing them is impossible! If our hard teeth can't puree them, our intestines don't stand a chance.

There are several exceptions to this (some pears and cherries, for example). We can eat the more tender skin of these fruits.

What about pesticides? Those are concentrated on the skin.

"But the skin contains the most vitamins! If we throw it out, we won't benefit from the nutrients!"

Let's not forget that fruit skins contain some vitamins and that only one-tenth of them would be enough for our needs, if only we could digest them.

The Combination of Fruit and Raw Vegetables

Is it possible to eat fruits with green salads and raw vegetables? Dr. Vetrano suggests eating lettuce with fruit to limit sugar intake.

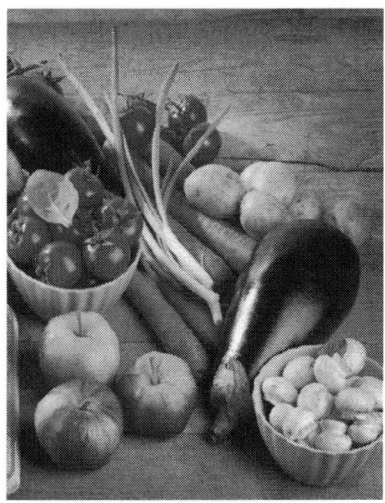

If our instincts were even the slightest bit functional, we would stop finding pleasure in food as soon as had an excessive serving of sugar. Alas, most of us have perverted, depraved instincts that don't function properly.

Therefore, we could easily eat raw vegetables after eating fruits.

To limit sugar, one can certainly have a large tomato with fresh fruit, but not more, due to the oxalic acid it contains.

Raw vegetables and greens can also be seasoned with citrus juice, avocado, and yogurt. A bit of parsley is also acceptable, as is a bit of moderately salted cheese crumbled atop the salad. No spices, no salt, and no other seasonings.

Fruit and Cooked Vegetables

Can we eat fruit before or after eating cooked vegetables?

The acidity in fruits creates an obstacle for the digestion of cooked foods because they stop the production of ptyalin, an enzyme necessary for the first phase of starch digestion.

All vegetables contain at least a bit of starch, especially potatoes.

If you eat a single fruit, it's important to wait a while before eating cooked vegetables.

If you'd like to have a fruit after eating cooked vegetables, you must wait until the digestion of those vegetables has finished.

Partial Indigestion

Someone countered me by saying that the body would reject what it was unable to digest and that it there couldn't be any harm in that.

I would respond by saying that the problems it causes are easy to understand. In fact, the loss of gastric juices presents a huge loss to the body. These juices are not supposed to be lost. They are meant to be reabsorbed. They are as precious to the body as sperm, and their loss impoverishes the body. We can see this in a person with diarrhea. They no longer have the strength they had before the diarrhea. On the other hand, an individual who is fasting will feel stronger than the person with diarrhea or dysentery.

Moreover, indigestion leads to fermentation which produces alcohol and carbon dioxide which poison the body.

To know if we have totally or partially digested our food, we simply need to look at the state of the stool that follows. They should:

- be formed
- come in small quantities
- be odorless
- pass quickly
- not smear and stain the body
- pass without gas

Most people have foul-smelling, bulky stools and gas so horrible that it would make an army of assailants flee.

Fruit Tarts and Pies

We have discussed the effects of mixing fruit with starch. A single taste of acid destroys the ptyalin that starch digestion requires.

This is why fruit cakes and fruit tarts are indigestible. Apple pies, cherry tarts, and strawberry tarts, like all other cakes we add fruits too, are indigestible. If the fruit has been candied, it is twice as indigestible.

In fact, these cakes contain three incompatible ingredients:

- starch
- sugar
- acid

Therein lies two incompatibilities: starch/sugar and starch/acid.

Fruit and Yogurt

It is possible to eat fresh fruit with unsweetened yogurt, but if the yogurt is sweetened, it will no longer be compatible. Sweetened yogurts and fruit, much like sweetened fruit compotes, contain incompatible sugars which are digested differently by the body.

> ***Notes from the Publisher:*** *In the early days of Natural Hygiene, following Shelton's lead, some dairy products were tolerated, even though they went against the theory of what constituted the natural diet of human being. Mosseri allowed some crumbled, non-fermented cheese on salads, but only because he lived in France and without this compromise, his followers would have completely given up on the diet. Yogurt, being easy to digest, was also tolerated for the same reason. Nowadays, it's possible to find these products made without animal milk, so Mosseri's food combining rules would apply to them in the same way.*

Fruit With Milk

Children may drink milk until they are 7 or 8 years old. Adults, on the other hand, can't digest milk at all.

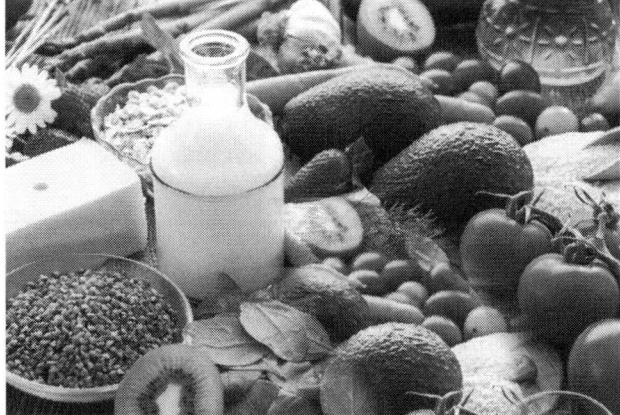

Children can handle this mixture without a problem because they have glands in their stomach that secrete renin, an enzyme that is necessary to digest milk.

When the child turns 7 or 8 years old, this gland atrophies and no longer secretes this enzyme. Thus, adults cannot consume milk.

The same goes for cattle which like renin.

Adults who drink milk, whether accompanied by fruits or curdled by citrus, will notice their stools becoming loose, yellowed and foul-smelling. The liver will quickly become overburdened leading to headaches.

Adults are better off abstaining from milk. Curdling milk with acids, such as those contained in fruits or citrus, has nothing to do with the process that occurs naturally due to the bacteria in milk or calf renin. The latter produces bacteria which is not what happens in the former.

Lastly, watermelons and other melons are incompatible with milk.

FRESH FRUIT	
COMPATIBLE WITH	INCOMPATIBLE WITH
Other fruits Greens Raw vegetables Dried fruits Yogurt	Watermelon and other melons Starches (potatoes, etc.) Cooked vegetables.

Watermelon and Other Melons

Watermelons and other melons are not acidic; they're neutral.

They're incredibly rich in water along with a particular kind of sugar that is very easy to digest but can rapidly ferment if its digestion is slowed in the small intestine.

When we buy these fruits, it's impossible to know in advance if they are going to be sweet or bland and tasteless. Therefore, it's tempting to add sugar when we eat them, but be careful!

This mixture of sugar and melon is indigestible. In fact, even if the fruit is bland, it still contains a bit of natural sugar, but it isn't the same kind of industrial sugar that we're tempted to add to it. The digestion of the first sugar is detrimental to the digestion of the second due to the different ways in which they are absorbed. As a result, the sugars ferment.

Remember that fermentation is guaranteed to occur when sugar is added to any fruit as we are often due with strawberries, grapefruits, pineapple, orange juice, etc.

I've noticed that citrus juices with added sugars typically cause heaviness and burping.

You only have to try this once to be convinced that it's true. The state of your stools the next day will be all the proof you need.

Though we can never be confident that watermelons and other melons are going to be sweet when we buy them, I've found that buying very ripe fruits is the safest bet. This isn't true for watermelons, however, as they become inedible if they are too ripe.

This is why watermelons and other melons are incompatible with other fruits. Because they are so rich in water, the excess water will disrupt digestion.

Watermelon and other melons are also incompatible with milk, yogurt, vegetables, potatoes, fresh fruits, dried fruits, and cheeses.

When these fruits are eaten with milk, it's too many liquids at one time. The stomach finds it much easier to separate liquids from solids than liquids from other types of fluids. When consuming melons with milk, it's impossible to segregate them. They thwart one another's digestion. One wants to pass through the intestines rapidly and be absorbed quickly while the other curdles and prefers to spend more time in the stomach in order develop. The pylorus won't open until the digestive curdling has completed, and by that time, the melons will have begun to ferment.

In conclusion, we can eat watermelon and other melons before any food, so long as we allow enough time afterward for them to be digested. For example, if we have a single slice of melon, we can eat other foods approximately ten minutes later, but if we have the entire melon, it's better to wait for an hour before eating something else.

CHAPTER 8: Dried Fruit

We include:

- Dates
- Dried figs
- Dried apricots
- Raisins
- Dried apple slices
- Dried pear slices
- Dried peaches
- Dried bananas
- Prunes
- Dried cherries

All these dried fruits are excellent for our health, except for prunes. They have a reputation for having laxative qualities. They are expelled by our intestines because they contain an acid that the liver can't oxidize.

Dates

There are two kinds of dates: dates on branches or dates with added glucose. The latter is soaked in glucose to prevent humidity from penetrating them and to allow for better conservation. This preservation technique doesn't seem to be too harmful because the layer of glucose that surrounds the date is very thin.

> **_Note from publisher_:** Nowadays you can find many types dates that have not been soaked in glucose.

Raisins

Raisins are soaked in paraffin for the same reason that dates are soaked in glucose: to prevent humidity from penetrating them. It's important to make sure to wash them before eating them by rubbing them with your fingers. Just rinsing them under running water is not enough.

Soaked raisins and their juice can be added to salad and raw vegetables.

They are an excellent replacement for sugar in yogurt.

Dried Bananas

Dried bananas that are sold in stores are excellent, but they have typically lost their natural fragrance because they've been sitting on a shelf for several months. If you dry the bananas yourself, they'll exude their marvelous banana flavor.

Here are the steps for drying bananas:

Buy extremely ripe bananas with blackish skin. They're usually sold at half-price. Peel them and arrange them on a platter in direct sunlight. Bring them in at night. After several days, they should be dry to the touch. This is only possible, of course, if the sun is intense, such as during the summer. In winter, the bananas can be placed in front of a heat source like a radiator or a fireplace.

Dried Figs and Apricots

Dried figs can be soaked in a bit of water which you can then drink. The dried fruits will inflate and become delicious. With a bit of cream, it can rival even the best cake!

In my experience, apricots are better dried than soaked.

When Should We Eat Dried Fruits?

Dried fruits are only compatible with a few foods. Shelton advocates eating them with a few moderately acidic fruits (apples, pears) or by themselves.

Nevertheless, I find that if they are eaten alone, there is a tendency to overeat them and do yourself harm. In fact, I have known many people who have been unable to stop themselves from eating large quantities (20 to 30 dates or 10 to 15 figs).

This is why I do not suggest eating them alone. I advocate for eating them only as a dessert, an hour after finishing a meal.

Dried fruits can be eaten in moderation immediately after eating fresh fruits to avoid having an excess of sugar. Personally, I prefer to eat my fill of fruits and not eat sweet dried fruits at all, but to each their own.

Abusing sugar leads to grogginess, heaviness, fatigue, low spirits, and lethargy.

Is it ok to eat sweet dried fruits with yogurt? Absolutely. People who enjoy eating sweetened yogurt will enjoy eating it with sweet dried fruits instead. They are much better than sugar and honey which are harmful to our health. The dried fruits can be cut into small pieces and be sprinkled on top of the yogurt, or mixed in it.

A Recipe

Is it okay to eat dates with raw vegetables? It seems okay to do so. In fact, it's the preferred salad of Iranian Natural Hygiene author, Hovanessian. Here are the ingredients:

- Lettuce
- Cucumber
- Carrots
- Tomatoes
- Fennel
- Celery
- Parsley

Cut all of the ingredients into small pieces and top the mixture with sweet dried fruits, such as dates and figs, that have also been cut into small pieces.

Hovanessian allowed honey in this salad, but I would advise against it. Honey is worse for us than white sugar! We steal honey from bees, so it should come as no surprise that it's harmful.

As a Dessert

Is it okay to eat sweet dried fruits after a meal of cooked vegetables or potatoes? Yes, but it's important to wait 30 to 60 minutes for the meal to be fully digested.

For Children

Is it okay to eat dates or other dried fruits with milk? It's not okay for adults, but it's perfectly fine for children. Dates can be crushed and added to warm milk.

Sweet Dried Fruit

COMPATIBLE WITH	INCOMPATIBLE WITH
Fresh fruits Yogurt Raw vegetables As a dessert at least one hour after a meal of vegetables or potatoes	All other foods Avocados White cheese

CHAPTER 9: Greens and Raw Vegetables

There's a movement in the United States that recommends exclusively eating fruit. In one of my books, I quoted several people who adhere to this fruit-only diet and remain satisfied and even enchanted with it as much as 17 years after starting.

The fruitarian diet is led by T.C. Fry, a relatively new Natural Hygienist to the professional scene. One of his arguments is the result of experiments conducted on gorillas at the San Diego zoo (as we know that people and gorillas are closely related).

The gorillas at the zoo were given a choice between fruits and greens, yet they continuously chose fruit throughout the entire experiment, which lasted all summer. They neglected the greens.

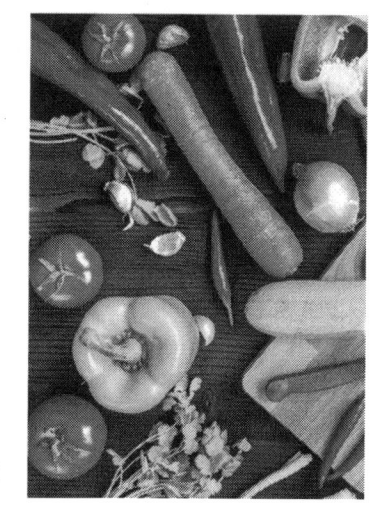

However, I learned that a Japanese zoologist observed gorillas living on a reservation in northern Japan in a harsh, snowy winter climate. These gorillas willingly chose to eat greens and raw vegetables, even when they were offered fruits.

Thus, we see that gorillas tend to prefer fruits in the summer and greens and raw vegetables in the winter.

I've also noticed that in the story of the Bible, when Adam and Eve were exiled from the Garden of Eden, God ordered them to live off greens and raw vegetables. Paradise is radiant health whereas illness is representative of purgatory.

This goes with my observation that chronically ill people would do better by eating more vegetables than fruits.

Therefore, healthy people can eat 70% fresh fruit and 30% greens, vegetables and potatoes. Ill people, on the other hand, should limit themselves to 30% fruits and eat 70% greens, vegetables, and potatoes.

We can most likely live on fruit alone (as many people already do), but it's also easy to abuse fruit by not respecting the rule that hunger should always precede our consumption of them.

Furthermore, overeating fruit can lead to:

Eating to Live Without Disease   by Albert Mosséri

- Frequent urination, day and night
- Partial insomnia in the middle of the night
- Tooth decay
- Abscessed teeth
- Restlessness

We should also note that, from a biological point of view, cucumbers, peppers, and tomatoes are also fruits since they have flowers.

SEASONINGS	
FORBIDDEN	**PERMITTED**
Vinegar Mustard Spices Salt Fresh onion Fresh garlic Fermented cheeses	Citrus Unsweetened yogurt Black olives Parsley Onions (sliced the day before) Slight salted and crumbled white cheese

People who are accustomed to eating greens and raw vegetables with salt, vinegar or mustard can replace these harmful substances with yogurt, citrus, black olives, mayonnaise or lightly-salted unfermented white cheese.

Raw vegetables are compatible with dried fruits, such as dates, dried figs, dried or cooked bananas and raisins. These fruits can be cut and mixed into a salad with raw vegetables.

A Salad Recipe

This dish should be eaten in the afternoon or a bit before the evening meal. Otherwise, it should be eaten before sleeping.

The following raw vegetables should be cut into small pieces and mixed into a salad:

- Lettuce or escarole
- Cucumber
- Celery
- Tomato
- Red pepper
- Chicory

Season with:

- Citrus
- Sliced black olives
- Onion (sliced the previous day so that it loses its spiciness)
- Olive or nut oil
- Parsley and chives, freshly picked

Optionally, oil can be replaced with

- Raisins or dried figs, cut into small pieces
- Dates without cores
- Fig juice (collected the day before)
- Maple syrup

The Presentation of Raw Vegetables

You have to be able to arrange raw vegetables on a plate in such a way that they're nice to look at and tempt people to gravitate toward them more than fruits or cooked meals.

I once knew a young Austrian woman who made amazing art with nothing but cut carrots, lettuce, fennel, parsley, tomatoes and other raw vegetables. She created designs in the form of a heart, the outline of a tree, and initials. The people who were fasting under my supervision were all enthralled, amazed and enchanted by what she did with vegetables.

Children especially appreciate such presentations and will enjoy preparing raw food art; This teaches them to make healthy food choices from a young age.

I know many Natural Hygiene practitioners who never managed to teach their children Natural Hygiene practices. Art with food is one way of teaching them to distance themselves from the bad habits of their little friends who eat sandwiches.

If they'd like, children may drink warm milk with raw vegetables, so long as they drink the milk first. These foods are compatible.

Raw vegetables are also likely compatible with watermelon and other melons, but no experiments have been done, and I don't know anyone that has tried the combination. The most liquid food (i.e., the melon) should be eaten first. I don't believe that this would lead to any digestive issues. I have often eaten raw vegetables after fruits without any problems. This provides all the more reason to eat watermelon and other melons, especially if there is a period between eating the two foods.

Any food which can be appreciated raw should never be cooked, such as carrots, fennel, celery, red peppers, and lettuce.

In the beginning, it will be hard to eat many raw foods due to our habit of eating them cooked. In the end, however, it's possible to enjoy them so much that you can't-do without.

It's all a question of habit and personal mental growth. I'm certain that the use of approved seasonings can help with eating and appreciate raw foods. I enjoy eating raw, unseasoned salsify as it tastes like almonds. I also enjoy raw celery, which tastes like coconut, raw Jerusalem artichoke, which is delicious with the skin, and raw green beans, still in their pods, which are my favorite. Nevertheless, I always keep a salad bowl full of cut and seasoned raw vegetables in case I want them between meals or before bed. I only use the acceptable seasonings previously mentioned.

It's better to properly chew raw vegetables than to drink them as juice because juices pass through the digestive system so quickly that they can't be properly digested. Moreover, undigested cellulose cleans out the intestines while the part that is digested provides benefits to the body.

It isn't prohibited to drink raw vegetable juice from time to time. Some raw vegetables can even be mixed, such as carrot and celery juice or fennel and carrot juice.

When I make carrot juice, I always add back the pulp. It's delicious, especially when drizzled with a layer of cream and topped with raisins.

RAW VEGETABLES	
COMPATIBLE WITH	**INCOMPATIBLE WITH**
Starches (potatoes, etc.) Cooked vegetables Yogurt Avocado Watermelon and other melons Fresh and dried fruits	Don't go back and forth between fruits and vegetables. Finish eating one in its entirety before eating the other.

CHAPTER 10: Vegetables and Root Vegetables

LIST OF VEGETABLES	LIST OF ROOTS
Zucchini	Potatoes
Green beans	Carrots
Artichokes	Parsnips
Celery	Salsify
Chicory	Celery root
Cauliflower	Rutabaga
Cabbage	Jerusalem artichokes
Brussel sprouts	Sweet potatoes
Eggplants	Yams
Green and red peppers	Tapioca
Broccoli	
Gourds	
Pumpkins	

Attention: It's important to distinguish between vegetables and legumes. They are not at all the same thing. Legumes are grains with a high concentration of protein: lentils, soy, dried and shelled peas, green beans, chickpeas and dried beans.

Legumes were created by nature for reproductive purposes, not for consumption. They are very difficult to digest. They cause bloating and horrible gas.

Legumes and the roots mentioned above are digested in the small intestines, but their digestive process begins in the mouth with ptyalin secretion that transforms them into sugar.

However, the slightest amount of acidity in the mouth can both destroy ptyalin and inhibit its secretion.

Therefore, no fresh fruits should be eaten before, after or in conjunction with legumes. All fruits contain acids except for bananas, melons, and watermelons, which I will discuss in a separate paragraph.

To put it simply, all foods that contain even the slightest bit of starch should be separated from foods containing acid.

Nature itself does not mix starches and acids in the foods it creates.

Mothers who crush bananas (starch) in orange juice are unintentionally doing great harm to their poor children because they are ignorant of the consequences. If they were to later smell their child's stools, they would understand their error immediately.

Furthermore, some people advocate eating fruits before meals, but the acidity in fruits lingers in the digestive tube for a rather long period until the body can dispose of them.

Thus, if we eat a single fruit, we can have a starchy meal after 20 minutes, so long as the apple has been completely digested. Some people have a sluggish digestive system and must wait for an hour.

On the other hand, if we eat various fruits, we must wait one or two hours before eating any cooked vegetables. If a person's digestive system is prolonged, they should wait several hours.

Lastly, the habit of eating fruit at the end of the meal as a dessert replacement is terrible. The acidity in these fruits stops the digestion of starches in its tracks, as we have already discussed.

Fruit pies, such as apple and cherry pies, are completely indigestible because the fruits incorporated in them are not compatible with starches. When we eat these foods, they pass through our digestive system as stool they next day, even when they haven't been thoroughly and properly digested. This causes us to lose some of our precious digestive juices and leads to fermentation. Fermentation, as we have already discussed, is essentially the same as poisoning our intestines.

Only onion, cheese, Swiss chard and spinach tart can be eaten, but these should also be eaten in moderation.

Tomatoes are an acidic fruit, botanically speaking. We mustn't eat them with cooked vegetables or potatoes.

All vegetables are compatible with one another. It's possible to mix several varieties in a stockpot.

Cooked vegetables are compatible with greens and raw vegetables, but they are not compatible with tomatoes and citrus.

If you'd like to eat a dessert, it's important to wait an hour after eating a meal. Sugar prevents ptyalin from acting and can disrupt starch digestion.

We can, however, eat dessert (cooked bananas, dates, etc.) immediately after eating fruits.

VEGETABLES AND POTATOES	
COMPATIBLE WITH	INCOMPATIBLE WITH
All other vegetables and roots Raw vegetables Greens Avocado	Fruits Tomatoes Citrus Yogurt Curdling milk White cheese

CHAPTER 11: Nuts and Seeds

When we talk about nuts, we're referring to walnuts, almonds, hazelnuts, cashews, pecans, coconut, pumpkin and sunflower seeds, pistachio, pine nuts, and sesame.

In the early 20th century, the first practitioners of Natural Hygiene, such as Shelton, turned to plant-based nuts as a source of protein after eliminating meat, fish, cheese, and legumes from their diet.

They believed that they were making a right decision, but in reality, their dietary change was even worse than only eating meat. The nuts they were eating contain at least twice as much protein as meat. They contain more than that if you consider that we eat nuts raw while we eat meat cooked, which destroys some of its protein value.

Regardless, eating these foods in excess leads to considerable consequences for our health:

- Foul-smelling stool and gas
- Infection
- Tooth decay and abscesses
- Insomnia
- Skin diseases
- Weakening of the digestive system

When we consume nuts, our digestive system is markedly weakened. We are no longer able to digest fruits so consuming even the slightest amount of them will cause light diarrhea. After eliminating various nuts from my diet, I found that I was able to eat as much as two kilos of fruits without any diarrhea.

Shelton advised that we eat 130 grams of nuts each day, but he later died from a debilitating disease like so many others often do.

It's tempting to argue that nuts meet the three criteria which qualify something like an acceptable food; they're pleasant to smell, pleasant to taste and pleasant to see.

In fact, when I start to eat cashews, I can't seem to stop, but as soon as I eat them, I feel an intense thirst that lasts for hours.

This thirst is a sign of irritation and mucous membrane inflammation due to stomach acid secretions. Healthy food should never provoke thirst.

Who's pretending that our instincts are in perfect condition and functioning normally? Haven't we already determined that our instincts are perverted and depraved? They're no longer reliable and can no longer guide us to choose healthy food.

Gorillas, on the other hand, have much more reliable instincts, yet they refuse to eat nuts.

Our sense of smell would have us eat plums and prunes, yet these foods will just remain undigested. Prunes are essentially laxatives, yet our sense of smell hasn't managed to detect this fact, and we continue to eat them.

Practitioners of Instinctive Eating would have you believe that you should just rely on your sense of smell to choose raw foods. Our sense of smell has become depraved and perverted from our abuse of tobacco, coffee, and artificial foods. We can no longer distinguish good food from bad food.

Some people have entirely lost their sense of smell! How are we supposed to choose foods by our sense of smell if we lack the sense altogether?

Therefore, we discourage eating more than one ounce of nuts a day. A small quantity of coconut or avocado may not be harmful. Personally, if I eat even half of an avocado I become very thirsty, so I no longer eat them. A teaspoon of almond butter or tahini is acceptable.

Problems From Overeating Nuts

Frequent consumption of large quantities of nuts can cause the following problems in sensitive persons:

- Headaches
- Bad taste in the mouth after waking up
- Lack of appetite
- Grogginess and lack of concentration
- Frequent urination, especially at night (to eliminate the toxic byproducts these foods produce)
- Sensitivity to acidic foods
- Tension which prevents relaxation, even when lying down
- Depression, pessimism, and anxiety
- Cystitis
- "Constipation" (the colon will try to dispose of the waste several times each day because it can't tolerate even the slightest amount of acidic stool)

- Flatulence and bloating
- Hunger due to malnutrition

- Stimulation followed by fatigue
- Desire to sleep for longer periods of time
- Weight loss

When people with no dietary restriction eat a few nuts, these symptoms won't be immediately evident, yet nuts are incompatible with virtually every other food.

In Egypt, many cafés serve a beverage called "khoshaf." It's made by soaking small pieces of peeled almonds, raisins, dates, dried figs, prunes, hazelnuts, and walnuts in rose syrup, yet this drink is still less harmful than traditional Turkish coffee or wine.

Eastern cafés often serve natural yogurt (called curdling milk), which is healthier than beer and other drinks, and this natural yogurt can also be found in cafés in France.

> **Notes from the Publisher**: I have read all of Mosséri's book and he changed his mind a few times on nuts and seeds. At some point, he banned them completely but eventually went back to a more moderate approach. Shelton recommended eating four or five ounces of nuts every day, which is a very large amount. The limit with Mosseri is one ounce for most people. Young athletes can have more.

CHAPTER 12: Cheese

Shelton once wrote that "in France, people eat cheese" just as we might say that "in Gabon, people eat fish in the morning" or even "in Japan, people eat raw fish!"

It seemed strange to him that people eat cheese and that there are hundreds of varieties of it. Who wouldn't lose their head in front of such an array! This variety is the door which leads to abuse. In Egypt, I only knew of a total of 4 or 5 types of cheese.

When a person stops eating meat, she immediately looks for other foods which contain protein as a replacement: cheeses, nuts, and legumes. This is a mistake; the large primates which are most closely related to humans, such as gorillas, never eat foods with a high concentration of protein, yet gorillas are immensely strong. It's said that they have the strength necessary to kill a lion. Indigenous peoples trapped a gorilla in a cave with the help of a very heavy rock. He moved the rock with only a slight movement of his hand, clapped his hands together as if to shake off the dust and banged on his chest as a sign of victory!

Milk is a perfect food for babies, but around the age of seven, a child's body will stop producing renin, the enzyme that is necessary to curdle and digest milk. This is why milk and dairy products are not suggested for adults.

In fact, cheeses contain 15% protein. Children need this much protein as they are still growing, but adults have already finished their growth. Therefore, adults, like the gorilla, should only consume the 1% protein that is contained in fresh fruits and vegetables. When dried, these foods contain approximately 5% protein.

I have personally fallen into this same trap by abusing dairy products. I experienced difficulties digesting my food, bloating, headaches, unhealthy stools, unrelenting tension, a bad taste in my mouth when waking up, and I often felt feverish, even when I didn't have a fever. I had previously recommended dairy products in my writings because I didn't dare to remove them from an already rather strict diet.

For the time being, I have relegated white cheeses as an occasional treat rather than a daily indulgence meant to nourish the body. I only approve of them when they are lightly salted (or not salted at all) and crumbled in a salad.

Cheeses are divided into the following three categories.

CHEESES

FERMENTED	COOKED	FRESH WHITE
Camembert Roquefort Brie Muenster Goat Aged Cantal All aged cheeses, even if they are cooked or white Parmesan Bleu Saint-Nectaire	Gruyère Fresh Cantal Dutch Mimolette Gouda Comté Tomme Babybel Saint-Paulin Mountain cheeses Etc.	Very lightly salted, such as: Époisse Saint-Florentin Ricotta Rigotte etc. Unsalted: Natural Kiri Samos

Cheese is a milk product. Therefore, since adults are not meant to consume milk, adults should also, ideally, give up cheese.

According to Natural Hygiene practitioner T.C. Fry, the milk curdling process that's required to create cheese causes fermentation which putrefies the casein present in milk. Therefore, the end-product should be indigestible.

I have noticed when tasting cheeses that I only savor the first bite, and then, I feel nothing. When I eat fruits, raw vegetables or cooked vegetables, on the other hand, I enjoy every single bite. Try eating a single bite of gruyere by itself. Your second bite will then seem tasteless while the third will seem foul.

The taste of natural foods should be the same with every bite for us to appreciate them.

Fermented cheeses are catastrophic for our health. They ferment the entire food bolus and poison the body.

Cooked cheeses are less harmful than fermented cheeses. They can be crumbled over raw vegetables.

Unsalted or lightly-salted white cheeses are least harmful when eaten in small quantities, crumbled over a salad or eaten separately from other meals. One or two tablespoons are acceptable.

When eaten immediately after fruit, cheeses complicate digestion. The same is true of starches. It's important to wait a short while before eating even a small serving as a treat.

Cheeses are compatible with greens and raw vegetables. Otherwise, they should be eaten alone, separately from meals and only on occasion. They should not be eaten daily. Cheeses must also be eaten without sugar or honey, as honey is much more harmful than sugar.

CHAPTER 13: Milk

We've met several people, especially people from the countryside, who have come to us for treatment to rehabilitate a damaged liver. Detailed analysis of their diet immediately revealed a huge mistake: consuming large quantities of milk. Some people had been drinking a large glass each day; others had been drinking more. That was enough to destroy their liver, give them jaundice, headaches, liver spots, gas and foul smelling, loose stools. Their digestive power was also damaged. When waking up in the morning, their mouth tasted pasty or bitter.

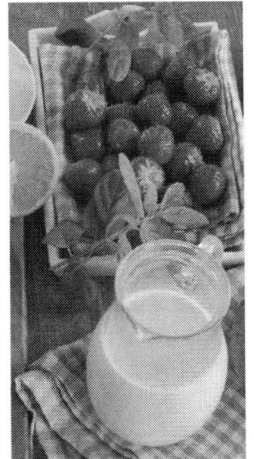

In reality, adults are incapable of digesting milk and other dairy products: custards, sweetened creams, ice cream, pudding, lattes, milk chocolate, etc. Not only is milk indigestible, the sugar that is often added to it further complicate the complete digestion of foods.

Babies, on the other hand, can digest it because their stomach secretes renin which curdles milk. It's the same as a calf's milk digesting enzyme, which is absent in adult cows.

Of course, a bit milk is often added to pumpkin soup, and this is perfectly fine. Custard is also acceptable without sugar (raisins can be used in place of sugar; artificial sugars are extremely toxic). Children can eat custard as a dessert from time to time, but there should be no other exceptions to the rule. Coffee, tea, and cocoa should never be consumed. These drinks are prohibited.

Milk should be given to babies and children until they are 7 or 8 years old. More milk should be given to babies than to children. In fact, at five years of age, the quantity of milk and dairy products a child consumes should be much lower than when they were toddlers. As we have already discussed, consumption of milk should have stopped completely by 7 or 8 years of age.

All species which nurse their offspring cut them off at a certain point in their development. No person is nursed into their old age! Unable to nurse from their mother's breast, people turn to cow, goat and sheep milk.

Children should be nursed by their mother until around three years of age. If the mother does not nurse her child (a grave mistake), the child should be fed by a wet nurse or, in the worst case scenario, cow's milk.

If the child is to be given cow's milk, it should be warmed, skimmed and diluted before being consumed. The milk must never be boiled. Raw milk is perfectly healthy. It's sometimes sold in grocery stores. What about microbes, you ask? It's the terrain that matters, not the microbes. Furthermore, we encounter microbes everywhere, even in the air we breathe.

Microbes can be useful for our bodies, such as our intestinal flora. They allow for cellulose digestion, protein synthesis, and processing of certain rare vitamins such as vitamin B1 and B12.

For children, milk is compatible with fruits, vegetables, potatoes and dried fruits.

Children often enjoy warm milk with crushed dates or a fig that has been soaked and softened the day before. They also enjoy custard prepared from raw milk and starch with raisins sprinkled on top. This is the famous Eastern "sahlab," flavored with cinnamon and rose water.

Rice pudding is acceptable for children as an occasional treat if the sugar is replaced by soaked raisins and the pudding is accompanied by the highly sweet water used for soaking.

White chocolate is primarily made from powdered milk. It can replace regular dark chocolate which often makes children agitated and nervous due to the abundance of theobromine it contains.

Milk cannot be consumed with watermelon and other melons. These foods are very liquid and elicit a very different digestive response.

MILK

COMPATIBLE WITH	INCOMPATIBLE WITH
Fresh fruit	Avocado
Dried fruits	Watermelon and other melons
Raw vegetables	
Cooked vegetables	
Potatoes	
Yogurt	

CHAPTER 14: Chapter Meat, Fish and Bread

Influential French and German biologists have done comparative studies of the anatomy and physiology of all living species. They created a table which indicates that humans are neither carnivorous nor granivorous but non-granivorous vegetarians.

In reality, humans do not have the attributes necessary to hunt and kill prey and immediately consume it. We lack the claws, sharp teeth and digestive juices that are required for the digestion of meat.

People also lack the gizzard that birds possess to grind up any grains which they may peck and a sufficient quantity of ptyalin secreting glands which, as we've discussed, are necessary for starch digestion. Moreover, we must cook grains to eat them. No animal, other than human beings, cooks their food before eating it.

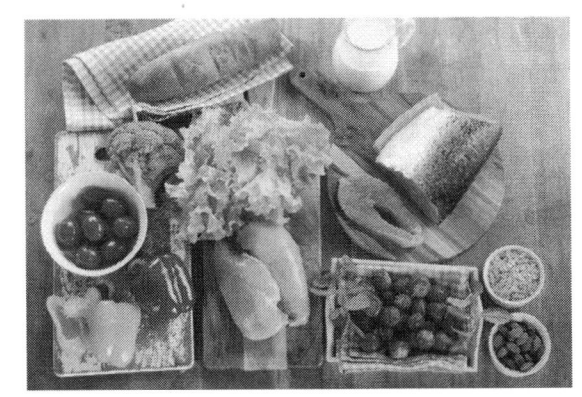

Normal, natural instincts would have us shy away from meats, but our instincts have become depraved and perverted to the point that we no longer taste anything. Instinctos, who rely on their instinct and sense of smell to choose foods, are making a major mistake in the way they make their choices.

It's true that cavemen had raw, gamey and rotting meat in their diet, but was that the typical diet for all of ancient human history?

On the contrary, for the majority of human history, people have lived in mild, tropical climates on a diet of fruits and greens growing naturally. Only a tiny fraction, lost in Europe and trapped by the cold, were forced to eat raw meat to survive. Cavemen, sick and out of control, inevitably vanished.

Another tiny fraction of people, lost in the North Pole in the ice and cold, had to eat raw fish to survive. These people were the Inuits, and they lived in complete misery for, on average, 27 years until their untimely death.

These aren't examples of diets we should follow, as the Instinctos would have you believe, but steps along the path to becoming extinct.

Children whose sense of taste has not yet been perverted don't like meat. Who could eat it in its natural state, without seasoning, without being cooked, without salt and sauce?

Who among us would kill a sheep or a chicken just to satisfy their hunger? Slaughterhouses are a disgusting sight.

Humans only recently began to eat meat in our 5 million years of history. At the beginning of time, humans were always vegetarians and foraged like gorillas rather than hunting or farming for food.

Legends of paradise all describe an earthly place in which people live in an orchard, eating the garden's delicious fruits, as in the Garden of Eden. All of these legends resemble one another. Isn't that strange? These tales don't describe this earthly paradise as being a horrific place of animal slaughter.

It's easy to say that these legends are nothing more than myths from the imagination of ancient peoples, but they are memories of ancient times, transmitted from generation to generation among the majority of earth's peoples, no matter how isolated and distant from other civilizations they may have once been.

Adam and Eve didn't eat bread or rice.

ILLNESSES BROUGHT ABOUT BY EATING MEAT AND HIGH-PROTEIN FOODS
Infection
Abscesses
Insomnia
Cardiac diseases
Cancer
High blood pressure
Skin diseases

ILLNESSES BROUGHT ABOUT BY BREAD AND GRAINS

- Common cold
- Sinusitis
- Bronchitis
- Catarrhs throughout the body
- Colitis
- Enteritis
- Rheumatism
- Gout
- Arthritis
- Sciatica
- Polyarthritis
- Lumbago
- Gallstones and kidney stones
- Partial insomnia
- Constipation

When you don't eat bread, you never catch colds! Experiment with this.

When I say bread, I also include grains, pasta and all products derived from flour, such as cookies, crackers, pancakes, cakes, pizzas, etc.

Chapter 15: Combining Bad Foods

When a new practitioner begins to eliminate various poisons (coffee, wine, tobacco, spices, etc.) and begins to change his diet in favor of a healthier way of life, they do so valiantly, courageously, and in spite of opposition from their friends and family. They do it because they have an important reason that's driving them.

In reality, the sometimes grave and precarious state of their health is a powerful motivation to change the course of their life and stick with the change.

When we're young, we're able to change much more easily because the body finds it easier to adapt and the mind has not yet become used to bad habits. Memories of various delicious tastes have not yet become anchored in their minds; they are not haunted by the past, whether pleasant or not.

Unfortunately, this is not the case for adults. After one or two years of a strict Natural Hygiene diet and knowing how to address the harmful effects of toxic foods, we eventually lose the fear of illness, and as a result, we might be tempted by the various desires plaguing us.

We need only watch TV, look at a store window, accept an invitation to go to a restaurant or sit in a café, read a magazine or speak with a neighbor to be assaulted by negative suggestions that directly or indirectly entice us to eat unhealthy foods.

How are we supposed to resist this attack when it comes at us from all sides, and we're already extremely tempted to taste the forbidden fruit?

We can't live in isolation, separated from society.

This is what leads us to deviate from a healthy lifestyle. Every hygienist does this at some point or another then return to their strict diet. Some skip the meal following their deviation while others fast for 24 hours, but very few manage to avoid committing these mistakes entirely.

With that being said, it's important to remember that as a rule of thumb, all deviations from a healthy diet are incompatible. Of course, there are rare exceptions, but the forbidden and harmful food will not be compatible with any other foods, no matter how healthy they may be.

Wine, Beer and Alcohol

Many hygienists stop drinking wine, beer and other alcoholic beverages but still indulge occasionally, especially when they are invited out with friends.

Others try to minimize their consumption of alcohol without eliminating it from their diet.

However, it's important to note that wine, beer, and other alcoholic beverages are incompatible with meals, regardless of whether or not they are healthy. When we drink wine with a meal, regardless of what the meal is, the food bolus will ferment. When the body rejects this bolus the next day, the stool will be bulky, nauseating, unformed and accompanied by foul-smelling gas. As a result, we won't profit from whatever we ate.

If we absolutely must drink wine, it's important that we keep it to a minimum. It must be consumed on an empty stomach. The same is true for beer and all other alcoholic beverages.

When given this advice, a practitioner will say, "Under those conditions, I'd rather not drink it at all!"

"That's for the best," I think to myself, remaining silent.

Coffee, Tea and Cocoa

Most practitioners have considerable difficulties eliminating coffee, tea and cocoa from their diet. I have talked about this elsewhere in my other writings.

Coffee is often consumed in the morning as a stimulant, to wake up, to have a clear mind in the morning and to be able to tackle any work we need to get done, but these drinks are not compatible with any meals, no matter what the meal. The poisons they contain delay or prevent digestion. Moreover, the sugar we frequently add to these drinks creates yet another obstacle to the production of ptyalin which, as we now know, is necessary for starch digestion. What can we do?

We have to try to get along without these drinks, but if you must drink them when you first start a Natural Hygiene diet, it's important to drink them on an empty stomach, separate from a meal.

It's better for the body to eliminate these liquids alone than to be forced to eliminate a partially digested food bolus along with them because of the poisons they possess.

Of course, it's also better to drink decaffeinated coffee and tea or drinks that taste like coffee but are made from roasted grains. You can find the latter in health food stores (GNC, Whole Foods, etc.)

Sweets and Pastries

Some people feel tempted by candies, chocolate, and cakes. Nevertheless, it's important to remember that sugar inhibits ptyalin secretion in the mouth which prevents starch digestion.

Moreover, white sugar is made up of different substances than the natural fructose we find in fruits. White sugar is not compatible with fructose. The time required to proceed through the various phases of digestion is different for each of these sugars, and white sugar prevents natural sugar from being digested.

These facts indicate that we shouldn't eat sweets with starches and fruits. They are incompatible foods.

It's best to cut out these foods entirely, but if that's not possible, they should be eaten on an empty stomach. They must not be eaten immediately before or after meals, even if those meals are healthy. The habit of eating dessert is unhealthy on its own, but if it can't be avoided, eat the dessert at least one hour after meals.

Some people think that they are doing well by baking cookies, cakes and pies at home with whole wheat flour, brown sugar, extra virgin olive oil and other natural equivalents to processed foods. Unfortunately, these ingredient replacements tempt us to believe that a cake made at home is healthy and to indulge in it, but this isn't true.

I prefer people buying cakes and cookies from the nearest bakery. By purchasing the conventional desserts, we remove any doubt as to whether or not the foods are healthy.

Spicy Foods and Cured Meats

All cured meats and spiced foods inhibit digestive secretions. Furthermore, they induce faster peristalsis which tries to eliminate harmful food from the body as quickly as possible.

As a result, if we eat these spicy foods as part of an otherwise healthy meal, the healthy aspects will not be entirely digested. The entire food bolus will pass as stool the following day. We know that salt has weak laxative properties, and spices are even worse.

If you can't help being occasionally tempted by cured meats or spicy dishes, you must at least take care to only eat them in small quantities and to only eat them on an empty stomach, separated from other meals.

These foods are not compatible with anything.

Cheese, Meat, Fish, Eggs

When someone who is used to eating large quantities of these foods tries to eliminate them from their diet, it's normal to want to eat them from time to time. If that person is unable to overcome the temptation, they must nevertheless take care only to eat them in small quantities and not mix them with other incompatible foods. Incompatible foods include starches and proteins (i.e., cheeses and meats should never be combined).

Fermented, aged and spiced cheeses are forbidden.

Unsalted or lightly-salted white cheeses, on the other hand, can be eaten in small quantities and crumbled over a raw vegetable salad.

These foods can also be occasionally eaten with greens or vegetables, whether raw or cooked.

Bread, Rice, Pasta

Diets based on Natural Hygiene should avoid these foods, but again, some people have told me that they are occasionally tempted to eat them.

Those who are unable to resist these temptations altogether should only give into them on rare occasions, and when they do, they should eat as little as possible.

Under these conditions, bread, rice and pasta can be eaten with green salads and vegetables, whether raw or cooked.

However, these grainy foods are incompatible with all fruits and proteins.

TABLE OF INCOMPATIBLE MISDEMEANORS						
	Fresh fruits	Dried fruits	Yogurt	Raw vegetables	Potatoes	Cooked vegetables
WINE, BEER, ETC	No	No	No	No	No	No
COFFEE, TEA, COCOA	No	No	No	No	No	No
SWEETS	No	No	Yes	Yes	No	No
CURED MEATS	No	No	Yes	No	No	No

| GRAINS | No | No | No | Yes | No | Yes |
| MEAT, FISH, CHEESE, EGGS | No | No | No | Yes | No | Yes |

CHAPTER 16: What's Important and What's Secondary

It's important to be able to distinguish between what's important and what's secondary. In general, people attach the most importance to insignificant factors and ignore the factors that are vital.

We read diet books and make change several aspects of what we eat, but we don't bother to make the most significant changes.

This is why I keep repeating the things that are most important to remember.

For example, we insist on eating artificial foods, even when we have to take medicine as a result. We want to modify our diet to be healthier, but we continue to take pills and other chemical substances purchased from a pharmacy!

I refuse to give nutrition advice to people who are still taking drugs. There's no point in changing your diet if you're going to continue to poison yourself with concentrated chemical products like pills.

Thus, on a scale of what is most and least important, we must take care to give priority to the following things:

1. Eliminate all chemical poisons, medicines, and drugs from your diet.

2. Choose human-specific foods and progressively eliminate all other foods from your diet.

3. Do not eat unless you are truly hungry. Calm this hunger by eating a few fruits in several sittings.

4. Choose compatible foods.

5. Eat them in the state that Nature has given them to us (raw and unseasoned).

6. Eat only when you are in a good place, both mentally and physically. Eat only when you are in a good mood, are calm and are not experiencing any pain, fever or anguish,

James Thomson, a Scottish naturopath, and something of a Natural Hygiene practitioner, prioritized frugality in a diet of conventional but organic foods. He was undoubtedly inspired by Cornaro, an Italian aristocrat who lived to be 104 years old by eating only 700 grams of food each day and eating whatever he wanted.

I tend to see frugality as a negative attitude. It's natural to seek satiety from one's diet, yet if this state is achieved through modern foods, the body will suffer greatly. In reality, modern foods are highly concentrated. If we stuff ourselves with bread, meat, and eggs, we will quickly become ill.

Why not seek out foods that are intended for human beings rather than eating modern foods and then being forced to eat small portions and mitigate their adverse effects with medications?

When we wait until we are truly hungry to eat, the stomach shrinks and satiety is attained much more quickly. As a result, we can be fully satisfied while eating very little.

Primitive human beings didn't have kitchens, stoves, microwaves, dining rooms and cookbooks.

When ancient human beings were hungry, they gathered a couple of fruits and ate them then and there, beneath a tree.

This was the Garden of Eden. This was Paradise.

When changing diets, it's possible that you'll feel several symptoms, depending on whether the change was for the better or, the worse.

If the new diet is equivalent to the former diet (i.e., it is just as good or just as bad), you won't feel any symptoms at all.

An inexperienced person can neither interpret nor characterize these symptoms as right or wrong.

When these symptoms arise during a fast, it is even more difficult for an inexperienced person to understand them. Should they be worried by these symptoms and stop the new diet? Should they ignore the symptoms and continue? Sometimes it's dangerous to persevere, and sometimes it's dangerous to stop. An inexperienced person cannot possibly know the difference, and there is no single experienced Natural Hygiene practitioner who is always right because there is always a possibility of making a mistake.

However, if the new diet is worse than the previous diet, the person will experience problems which can easily be attributed to the diet and can easily be classified as good or bad.

If on the other hand, the new diet is better than the former, it's easy to misinterpret the problems that may arise. It's much harder to interpret them, attribute them to the diet and classify them as good or bad.

With that being said, some nutritionists are worse than the inexperienced person that is changing their diet. They express opinions that are completely misguided, foolish and unreasonable.

That's the driving force behind the screwed up system of Instinctive Eating. Those who follow this stupid system end up with massive hair loss originating from malnutrition, but Guy-Claude Burger would have practitioners believe that it is just part of the detox!

As though hair loss was just a detox symptom! What can we say in the face of such nonsense? The person behind it must have his head in the clouds.

This is absolutely a negative symptom which proves that the diet in question is causing malnutrition. Hair loss can also occur when a fast has been pushed to unsafe limits. It is a negative symptom which cannot be classified as a good thing.

Instinctotherapy practitioners consume cassia, a vegetable-based laxative, with every meal; they eat large quantities of various nuts. These are both serious mistakes which diminish our body's digestive power and lead to malnutrition and hair loss.

Let's look at a positive example, on the other hand. A practitioner adopts a healthy diet without any stimulants, coffee, alcohol, spices or highly-concentrated proteins. This practitioner immediately begins to feel extreme fatigue. This symptom is worrisome for the practitioner, but in reality, it's a helpful, positive sign.

The meaning behind the symptom is significant as it has the power to either encourage or discourage the new practitioner.

Moreover, it reveals whether the practitioner is on the right track or is in a downward spiral. It explains if changes need to be made or if the practitioner should only persevere.

Is weight loss associated with diet change positive or negative? Is it a good thing or a bad thing?

Are the stimulation and euphoria felt after eating certain foods good or bad?

Only a highly experienced Natural Hygiene practitioner can give a qualified opinion. The professional will know whether or not the practitioner's health will be improved or worsened by the symptoms.

Here's an example is taken from a reader of Healthful Living, a publication in the USA.

> "One of your articles,: writes a reader, "spoke of a young man who ate everything raw when he was home."
>
> "He left for military service and ate the same food as everyone else at the table, as they say.
>
> "As a result, he experienced a series of issues with his health.
>
> "In the end, as soon as he returned home, he returned to his diet of raw foods and once again found the health he had once known.
>
> "You used this story," wrote the skeptical reader, "to illustrate and praise raw food diets, this fad, this far-fetched way of life.
>
> "But if the body had been raised on this type of diet, it's normal that the poisons present in today's foods would be detrimental to it.
>
> "Those who rapidly switch to your diet, on the other hand, will also experience these same issues with their health and these same illnesses, though they may not be as marked.
>
> "I'm trying to say that any sudden change, for better or worse, will result in illness.
>
> "Therefore, we can't conclude that the soldier's return to his raw vegetable diet is proof that this diet is the best thing."

Fry, a Natural Hygienist, responded:

> "You say that the dramatic changes that take place in the body are pathogenic, but you're only partially correct.
>
> "In reality, if a person changes their diet to foods that are toxic, as cooked foods are, you are correct, but if the individual is beginning to eat raw foods, you are incorrect, even if pathological symptoms arise.
>
> "In the first case, the body shows symptoms because it still possesses enough vitality to reject the toxins that result from cooking, such as coagulated proteins and caramelized starches.
>
> "In the second case wherein a person changes their diet to eat raw foods, the body's vitality improves, and it begins to reject toxic substances that weren't eliminated in the past. This is why I say you're only partially correct."

Good or Bad?

For more clarity, we've seen that illness can mean one of two things:

- the person is on the right track
- the person is on a downward spiral

It's up to the professional Natural Nygienist to decide this. An inexperienced practitioner is incapable of judging. Let's look at an example:

A person stops drinking coffee and experiences headaches.

Another person who never drinks coffee has one or two cups and also experiences a headache.

Both people have headaches, but the first is on the right track and is experiencing detox symptoms. The second person is experiencing headaches because the coffee is poisoning them.

Allow me to make a small digression. Fry considered cooked foods to be toxic, yet this depends on how the food is cooked. Prolonged cooking in oil or butter with added pepper, wine, sauces and other aromatics is certainly very harmful.

With that being said, medicines, coffee, tobacco, fermented cheeses (recognizable by the thin, whitish crust that covers them, powdered with mold) and wine are much more harmful than cooked foods.

There are certainly some types of cooking which are acceptable and pose almost no risk of harm: rapid cooking at a low temperature with water instead of fat. It is a sort of semi-cooking technique. Let's not forget that the people of New Guinea work vigorously, yet they live for an extended time eating a diet composed 90% of sweet potatoes cooked over hot stones.

Fried foods, on the other hand, are the worst foods out there.

CHAPTER 17: Natural Combinations

In nature, we see that foods are made up of many different elements. For example:

1. Fresh, ripe fruits, such as apples, pears, oranges, etc. contain:
   - sugar
   - acids
   - small amounts of protein
   - no starches (unless they are green fruits)
2. Green leaves, vegetables and roots contain:
   - carbohydrates
   - small amounts of protein
   - no acids

Notice that these natural foods do not contain mixtures of acids and starches.

Even if we enjoy eating apples with oranges due to the pleasure this combination brings, we're not allowed to eat oranges with starches.

Nature has shown us what to do; we mustn't go against her.

One of the most common criticisms of compatible foods is that Nature herself has mixed various elements in natural foods. For example, wheat contains both starches and proteins.

The following elements, however, are not mixed in natural foods:
1. acids and starches
2. starches and sugars
3. various proteins in a single food
4. various starches in a single food
5. fats and acids
6. sugars and concentrated proteins

It is true that there are natural foods which contain sweet starches, such as sweet potatoes, chestnuts, and bananas.

Thus, in general, Nature gave us guidelines through the dosage of elements that she artfully composed. Nature separated certain elements to avoid impeding their digestion. Eating everything pell-mell disrupts Nature's perfect order.

What is Nature's correct design? All animals have a monotonous diet, year-round. In the wild, dogs are content with their carnivorous diet; birds are primarily granivorous. These animals don't partake in the immense variety of foods that humans spread across their tables.
Thus, as a rule, we must try to follow Nature's example in her natural combinations.

Foods that are identical or nearly identical in composition (i.e., most fruits) can be eaten together without a problem.

Foods with very different compositions, on the other hand, are better off being separated.

Thus, we don't need scholarly explanations or familiarity with chemistry to be able to nourish ourselves healthily.

"In general, most foods contain starches, proteins, and fats," writes Fredericks. "This is what makes Dr. Hay's diet somewhat misleading."

Dr. Hay especially emphasized the incompatibility of starches and proteins. He fed his patients starches and proteins in separate meals to avoid any problems which might arise, in reality, from excessive portions of protein.

"He borrowed this rule from hygienists," says Shelton, "and paid very little attention to other Natural Hygiene rules concerning food compatibility. Therefore, I suppose Fredericks was addressing this disassociation of protein and starches.

"If he believed that this disassociation was misleading, it is merely because he wasn't paying enough attention to the digestive process.

"It's true that Nature has created such combinations, but these foods are natural and are therefore not difficult to digest.

"As a result (and this fact is ignored by most dieticians), the body is able to adapt its digestive secretions – in terms of acids, its enzymes and their settling time – to the needs of the food in question, while such a precise adaptation of gastric juices isn't possible when two completely different foods are consumed."

Human-Specific or Compatible?

We find that this argument over artificial and natural food combinations is far-fetched.

Why? Because the grains and legumes involved in this argument are not meant to be consumed by human beings!

Don't grains contain both proteins and starches?

Shelton's response might be valid for the birds that eat these foods, but it's undoubtedly irrelevant for human beings as we are not meant to consume grains.

Who said that grains were easy to digest? They aren't.

When we eat whole wheat bread, whether by itself or with a bit of cheese, digestion will always be delicate, with some differences, depending on whether or not the bread was consumed alone.

What's interesting is that rather than eliminating bread and even cheese, instead of seeking to make their digestion less difficult – something wholly hypothetical and illusory – we aim to mitigate their effects.

Bread is not food that is meant to be eaten by human beings. It will always lead to digestive difficulties whether it's salted, whole wheat or consumed in conjunction with compatible foods by the Sheltonian school of thought.

No compromise will make bread acceptable for the human body. These accommodations are merely a lesser evil.

The specific nature of natural foods should take precedence over their compatibility in all discussions and considerations concerning their quality, and whether or not they are acceptable for human consumption.

How does Nature combine starches and proteins? Roots contain a lot of starches and very few proteins. Vegetables and greens contain very little protein and very little starch.

High-Protein Foods Distort the Problem

In *Hygienic Review,* vol. 37, no. 1 (September 1975), Shelton published a fascinating article by Dr. Ralph Bircher Benner on the controversial question of proteins.

> "Kofranji, of the Max Planck Institute, proved that it is possible to maintain a balance of protein consumption and excellent physical performance by consuming only 25 grams of protein each day.
>
> "On his side, Oomen and Hipsley found a population that succeeded in developing both magnificent health and incredible musculature and physical performance while eating nothing more than 15/20 grams of protein each day,"

This is what routs all dieticians.

I don't see why Shelton and so many others have recommended such high doses of protein. With too much protein, health problems are inevitable. These problems cannot be blamed on lousy food combinations!

COMPOSITION OF HIGH-PROTEIN FOODS

Foods are classified as high-protein when they contain a high percentage of proteins (10% to 50%). Examples of these foods include:

- Nuts, hazelnuts, cashews, almonds, pistachios, pumpkin seeds, sunflower seeds, etc.
- Meat, fish, poultry, cold cuts.
- All kinds of cheese.
- Eggs.
- Oysters and other shellfish.
- Legumes (dried peas, white beans, chickpeas, lentils, dried beans).

In nature, there are no foods that only contain pure protein.

Foods that contain only a bit of protein are not classified in this example. Examples of these foods include:

- Avocado, black olives.
- Fruits and vegetables, including roots.

Foods that are rich in protein are not meant to be eaten by humans and create considerable digestive problems which make them too strong and harmful.

Gorillas, which are related to humans, do not eat these foods, yet this doesn't stop them from having impressive musculature, tremendous strength, and power which makes human beings seem really weak, as though they were a lesser species on the brink of extinction.

Natural combinations of high-protein foods don't concern us because the high-protein foods themselves don't affect us.

The Digestion of Natural Combinations

> "Digestion," writes Shelton, is a physiological process in which the body changes up its activities to suit the various characteristics and needs of the food that is trying to process into usable materials.

> "A remarkable fact may be noted regarding the work carried out by digestive glands: namely, the digestive system can change its fluids and enzymes to adapt to the characteristics of the foods we eat.

"To this end, let's look at this quote from Arthur C. Cuyton in his classic Textbook of Medical Physiology (Second Edition, 1961):

"In certain portions of the gastrointestinal tract, the types of enzymes and other secretions change in relation to the types of food that are present."

"Pavlov undoubtedly further emphasized the digestive tract's ability to adapt its fluids and enzymes to the type of food being consumed though we already had some knowledge of this fact before his notorious research.

"Let us note in passing that physiologists today know these facts, but neither Pavlov nor any physiologists among them have tried to draw from this information a practical conclusion for everyday life. They haven't applied this knowledge in their daily diet. Physiology seems to be viewed as a "pure" science with no practical relationship with an individual's daily life.

"Variations in the components of digestive secretions, whether enzymic or otherwise, in accordance with an ingested food constitutes the body's effort to adapt its gastric juices to suit the digestive needs of various foods.

"These variations include changes in the alkalinity or acidity (pH) of secretions, the concentration of enzymes and their adjustment time, etc. to adapt to different foods.

"This adaptation of gastric juices and their enzyme levels to match the characteristics of ingested foods is not possible if the latter is composed of foods which are radically different from one another.

"These variations in the acid and alkaline concentration of secretions, their enzymatic composition and adjustment time can only take place if foods are eaten alone or with other foods which will not conflict with the digestive process that this category of food requires.

"Dr. Tilden used to say that Nature never produced a sandwich. It's clear that the human digestive system is adapted to the digestion of natural food combinations (i.e., those that Nature herself has combined), but it is surely not adapted to process artificial mixtures such as those that modern human beings eat every day."

Natural food combinations won't present digestive difficulties, so long as the foods in question are fit for human consumption.

Difficulties will arise, on the other hand, during meals made up of various incompatible foods, such as during Christmas feasts and other festivities. These celebrations tend to end up with an "epidemic" of mass poisoning.

The kind of artificial food mixtures that we eat today present an obstacle to any potential variation in digestive secretion composition which may be necessary to ensure proper digestion.

Therefore, we recommend only eating compatible foods to avoid these difficulties and conflicts in the digestive process.

It's all about respecting the limits of our enzymes.

We have repeated time and time that natural food combinations are easy to digest, so long as the foods in question are fit for human consumption.

If the food in question is not meant to be consumed by human beings (such as seeds, grains, and legumes), digestion will become difficult.

We already know how difficult it is for the human body to digest legumes. They lead to gas, foul-smelling stool, decreased energy, heaviness, bloating and long periods of digestion.

We must keep in mind that the distinction between a natural combination of foods fit for human consumption and artificial combinations of two or more foods which are also fit for human consumption has never been the subject of comparative experimentation.

Although Dr. Tilden was a professor of physiology at a medical school in the USA, he lacked confidence in physiologists.

"There's no reason," he would say, "to split hairs about the chemical composition of foods and stomach secretions nor is there any reason to cause a useless controversy. No one can be certain as to how the body reacts when foods are mixed in the stomach."

Dr. Tilden was at the forefront of progress being made in the field of food compatibility.

Therefore, we must stay as close as we possibly can to what is simple and logical to avoid making mistakes.

Chapter 18: The Natural Hygiene System

Some general concepts

Let's return to this correspondence between Mr. Fry, director of the American publication Healthful Living, and one of his critics, already quoted above:

> "Please excuse my overly harsh letter and my unproven condemnations, but your writings make my blood boil.
>
> "In conclusion, allow me to change my tune. Continue sending me your magazine. It's very different from other health magazines, but you can, all the same, do some good.
>
> "I would like to suggest that you write shorter articles and cut out useless information. Use tables and give biographies of your contributors. Give your sources on controversial subjects (which is practically everything you write!) and don't condemn all other outlooks in a single stroke of your pen. Deliver your message in concise, clear terms and try to change up your format.
>
> "Lastly, choose a theme for each issue and stick with it." – Paul J. Kleiber, Hilton Head Island, SC, USA

Our Origin

Here is the detailed response of magazine director, T.C. Fry:

> "In the study of nutrition, a scientific approach means determining our biologic origin and using it to determine our dietary characteristics. The rest comes from minor details.
>
> "For example, a horse can live a vigorous life and enjoy excellent health from birth to death on a diet of only grass and its mother's milk. It will be healthy, alert and fast until the day it dies. The same is true of gazelles and other creatures in nature.
>
> "Horses are herbivores and eat nothing else.
>
> "Yet, according to recent nutritional guidance, we should be omnivores, like pigs. According to modern thought, we should be carnivorous, granivorous, herbivorous, frugivorous, saprophytic and even insectivorous!
>
> "However, anthropology, biology, and physiology have all proclaimed that humans are frugivorous. They have said this for

more than two hundred years now. Classic texts and literature even taught this until the beginning of this century.

"The prostitution of scientific institutions to commercial interests, especially the meat and dairy industries, have led dietitians to pervert their knowledge.

"In fact, I've fought more than once with people who place a blind confidence in common mistakes rather than accepting the truth when they are confronted with it.

"As for readers who write us to explain their own experiences, they aren't always precise, but they reflect the good that can be drawn from our advice being put into practice.

"In short, when you characterize a raw food diet as a hobby, you are looking at things incorrectly. In fact, cooking is the real hobby! Almost everyone is victim to this pathogenic practice.

"In Nature, human beings ate raw fruits and nothing else. No one had stoves or microwaves. We ate only what captured our attention with its scent and flavor and consumed it for the pure pleasure of eating.

"To disagree with me, people often cite passages from the Bible about meat as food.

"Yet, it is my understanding that in the Bible, humans were placed in a garden, an orchard, not a menagerie! Moreover, no cooking devices were made available in this garden!

"Even if this story seems to be nothing more than a legend or unrealistic fable, it nevertheless paints a precise portrait of the human condition in favorable climates that existed until recent times.

"I would say instead that human beings were placed in neither an orchard nor a slaughterhouse.

Acute Illness

"Acute illnesses are triggered by the body to quickly detox and repair an infected body.

"These illnesses are brought about by ingested poisons and waste that has not been successfully eliminated, not the symptoms of the disease itself.

"These illnesses are not cured because the disease is the cure.

"A diet which doesn't pollute the body and healthy life practices like those we advise in the article you're critiquing do not cause toxemia, but toxemia is at the core of the illness.

"When you improve the condition of your body, it can profit from the accrued vitality to trigger a total cleanse of your body. This is what we call illness.

"It's true that the symptoms of this cleanse are disagreeable and can take the form of a cold, flu, asthma, sinusitis, skin ulcers, herpes, etc.

The Science of Natural Hygiene

Here are some of the salient points from which our Natural Hygiene philosophy has evolved:

- Health is normal and natural. Illnesses are abnormal and unnatural, so they are not necessary.
- We cannot obtain health through the use of medications because they are poisons and drugs.
- Illnesses are not preventable and cannot be because they only exist if there is a cause for them.
- Illnesses are natural healing processes.
- Health can only come from healthy life practices.
- An affected body is capable of repairing itself. Rehabilitation is an exclusively biologic process. The force that created such a superb being from a microscopic fertilized egg continues working until the day it dies. This force is enough to restore a body's health because this force is what created the health, to begin with.

Some clarifications are necessary to understand the six principles listed by Fry.

When Fry says that health is natural, he seems to be expressing a banality, a common idea. Medicine, on the other hand, teaches that the normal human state is disease. In fact, it speaks about the illnesses associated with childhood, menopause, puberty and old age as if each of these phases of life is absolutely and necessarily accompanied by health problems. Illness is not inevitable. It doesn't just happen for no reason.

When Fry says that we can't prevent illness, he's referring to vaccinations.

When Fry says that health can only come from healthy life practices, this is not a banality either. You can't have good health if you keep drinking wine and coffee, using spices and eating fried foods, even if you're vaccinated against every illness there is.

Poisons in Natural Foods

Let's continue with the reader that wrote a letter to Fry:

"Secondly, I take what you've said about vegetables with a grain of salt. Where did you get your information stating that vegetables and greens are harmful? They're foods! (We know that this American magazine is opposed to the consumption of greens and vegetables, considering that humans are frugivorous – A.M.)

"In fact, an appropriate amount of a good selection of vegetables coupled with a good understanding of said vegetables can be an immensely catalytic support for nutrition. They are also effective against stress and bad moods, and they lead to well-being."

Here is Fry's interesting response:

"Since human beings are frugivorous, they do not have the enzymes necessary to disintegrate the various compounds present in plants and grains.

"Every compound that we can't metabolize is poison in our body. For example, rabbits, which are herbivores, happily eat nightshade, but even the slightest bit of it would kill a human being.

"Practically all plants and grains are toxic in one way or another.

"I drove myself insane trying to find this reference which I offer to all of my readers.

"In the September 23, 1983, issue of Science, a magazine published by the American Association for the Advancement of Science, there is a study published by Dr. Bruce N. Ames, Director of Biochemistry at the University of California, Berkeley.

"In his study, he accuses practically all of the following vegetables of being poisonous and carcinogenic:

Mushrooms
Celery
Rhubarb
Spinach

Onions and garlic
Radish
Okra
Potatoes
All greens

"Vegetables are not natural foods for human beings. They are harmful whether raw or cooked, though the cooking process destroys the poisons along with any nutritive value the vegetables may have had.

"Plants do not provide catalytic support for nutrition because their useful compounds (vitamins, minerals, fats, proteins, and carbohydrates) are digested and absorbed, losing their identities.

"Insofar as they are not digested – and most plants contain indigestible compounds – the plant is toxic if these compounds are absorbed.

"For example, the allyl mutagen contained in garlic and mustard oil is indigestible. They are extremely toxic to cells. They easily penetrate tissues, skin, kidneys, etc.

"These substances are also found in onions, chives, shallots, mustard, grains, etc.

"Stalks and greens do not provide the elements which are essential for our nutrition: carbohydrates.

"The catalytic support you speak of is a medical effect, not a health effect. The toxic compounds in the plants we exalt are essentially no different from marijuana, opium, caffeine, etc." – T.C. Fry.

Nevertheless, we should differentiate between garlic, onions, shallots, mustard, turnip leaves and, on the other hand, potatoes, lettuce and all other edible vegetables that are neither spicy nor bitter.

The former contains considerable quantities of poisons while the latter only contain minimal amounts of poison and cannot be considered dangerous.

Let's not forget that there are people living in the mountains of New Guinea at an altitude of 2,000 meters who eat a diet that is 90% composed of sweet potatoes cooked on hot stones and 10% of fruits and greens. These people are nevertheless vigorous and carry out arduous physical labor without falling ill. They live for a very long time.

The acids contained in fruits, on the other hand, can be considered poisons. The body must neutralize and eliminate them before being able to profit from their nutritive substances.

Dr. Carlson seemed to support an idea like that of Fry's. He advised boiling vegetables three times to rid them of their mineral salts.

Are vegetables and greens toxic to the human body? I don't believe so.

Fry says that we cannot use gorillas as an example, for a while they do eat 90% greens, they do so because there is nothing else in their habitat. An experiment was carried out in the San Diego Zoo in the United States. It lasted all summer. Fruits and greens were both made available to gorillas for them to freely choose what they'd like to eat. They only ate fruits for the entire experience.

Nevertheless, I have been told from a trustworthy source that a Japanese zoologist found that during a rough winter in Northern Japan, gorillas who were faced with snow and extreme cold chose to eat greens and vegetables, despite being offered fruits.

Since we are more closely related to gorillas than to other monkeys which are lower on the evolution chart, we should use them as an example of how to live.

> *Note from the publisher:* The great apes are the most closely related animals to human beings, as Mosséri pointed out. However, he occasionally mentions that gorillas are the closest animal to our us. In reality, chimpanzees (and particularly bonobos) have been found since then to be the closest ape to human beings. That doesn't change much of what Mosséri says since chimpanzees eat fruits, vegetables, greens and minimal quantities of other foods.

Printed in Great Britain
by Amazon